EMOTIONAL EATING

The Secret Code for Recovery and
Ending your Lifelong Addiction

SIMON GRANT

© **Copyright 2019 by Simon Grant - All rights reserved.**

This document is geared towards providing exact and reliable information in regards to the topic and issue covered. The publication is sold with the idea that the publisher is not required to render accounting, officially permitted, or otherwise, qualified services. If advice is necessary, legal or professional, a practiced individual in the profession should be ordered.

- From a Declaration of Principles which was accepted and approved equally by a Committee of the American Bar Association and a Committee of Publishers and Associations.

In no way is it legal to reproduce, duplicate, or transmit any part of this document in either electronic means or in printed format. Recording of this publication is strictly prohibited and any storage of this document is not allowed unless with written permission from the publisher. All rights reserved.

The information provided herein is stated to be truthful and consistent, in that any liability, in terms of inattention or otherwise, by any usage or abuse of any policies, processes, or directions contained within is the solitary and utter responsibility of the recipient reader. Under no circumstances will any legal responsibility or blame be held against the publisher for any reparation, damages, or monetary loss due to the information herein, either directly or indirectly.

Respective authors own all copyrights not held by the publisher.

The information herein is offered for informational purposes solely, and is universal as so. The presentation of the information is without contract or any type of guarantee assurance.

The trademarks that are used are without any consent, and the publication of the trademark is without permission or backing by the trademark owner. All trademarks and brands within this book are for clarifying purposes only and are the owned by the owners themselves, not affiliated with this document.

Table of Contents

Introduction 1

Chapter One: What is Emotional Eating? 3
    What is Emotional Eating? 3
    Food Addiction 7
    Food Addiction vs. Emotional Eating.. 8

Chapter Two: Why Do We Eat? 13
    The Seven Classes of Food... 17
    Classes of Food/Food Groups.. 18
    Physical Hunger vs. Emotional Hunger... 30
    How does the brain signal physical hunger?............................... 32

Chapter Three: Emotional Eating and Well-being......................38
    Binge Eating Disorder 44
    Anorexia Nervosa 45
    What triggers anorexia in people?.. 46
    Emotional Eating in Children 49
    Emotional Eating in Adolescents 50
    Emotional Eating in Adults 50

Chapter Four: What is Emotion? 52
    The Subjective Component 53
    The Physiological Component 53
    The Behavioral Component 54
    Classification of Emotion 56
    Chemical Composition of Emotions 60

Chapter Five: Eating and Emotional Intelligence 68
    How to Identify and Express Your Emotions Properly 68
    What is emotional intelligence? 69
    Self-Perception Skills 70
    Self-Control Skills 73
    Social Perception 75
    Relationship Control Skills 78
    Emotional Regulation 81

Chapter Six: How to Deal with Emotional Eating 83
    General Acceptance 83
    Exercise 86
    Expressing your Emotions 87
    How to Tolerate Distress 94
    How to Practice Self-Connection 104
    Catching and Reframing Self-Defeating Thoughts 108
    Ways of creating empowering thoughts 111
    Develop New Core Beliefs 123
    Create a Support System 126
    Creating a support system at home 127

Creating a support system at work 129
　　Social Outings 130

Conclusion 135

Resources 135

Introduction

Food, water, and shelter… these are the three basic requirements for the survival of mankind on Earth. Deprivation of any of these three requirements will lead to the death of the individual involved. While food is absolutely necessary, man's attitude toward food has gradually changed and evolved over the years, and not for the better. Man has developed a lot of bad habits that are difficult to overcome. Habits like food addiction, emotional eating, anorexia, bulimia, and many more are experiences of the twentieth and twenty-first century.

This book is designed to help its readers overcome their problems with food. Determined to cater to needs of all, this book will help you recognize if you are an emotional eater, help you figure out why you do it, highlight the effects of it on your health (both mentally and physically), explain the impacts of it on your social life, and guide you on how to overcome the urges with the right mindset and level of control.

It contains the secret code and strategies you need to end that addiction, and every chapter is designed to take you a step closer to the end. The book was not created to teach you how to stop your terrible food relationship temporarily. The strategies highlighted and discussed in the chapters will totally redefine how you think about food. By now, you must be wondering what else you have to think about when consuming food, and that is the source of the problem. Food isn't just food; it has an important role to play in our lives, which isn't just something we eat. Read on to understand more.

Chapter One

What is Emotional Eating?

What is Emotional Eating?

Emotional eating can be defined as the binge consumption of junk, comfort food, and other unhealthy foods as a psychological response to the circumstances surrounding the individual. Circumstances in the previous statement could vary from experiencing traumatic accidents to achieving lifelong goals. Contrary to popular beliefs that people only eat emotionally when they are sad, it's also common to eat emotionally when you're happy. Imagine you are a top shot lawyer for one of the biggest corporate law firms in your state, and you were finally appointed as a partner in the firm after working there for ten years. Wouldn't you want to celebrate such an achievement? It would be odd not to. If you decide to celebrate with your friends and have a night of drunken revelry, emphasis on a single night, you're okay. It's good to appreciate and celebrate your victories in life. But the moment your first response to such news is to open your refrigerator and take out a pint of ice cream or order a large size pizza for your personal consumption, not because you're hungry but because you are happy, there is a problem. Eating large or unnecessary amounts of food as a response to the way you're feeling emotionally is a problem. Whether it's because you are sad or happy, it is a problem.

Your emotional situation should not justify the amount or the type of food you are eating.

Emotional eaters try to use the food to handle their emotions. They will keep eating subconsciously, not knowing that they have consumed an unnecessary amount of food. This is because they are not trying to satisfy their physical hunger. They are trying to satisfy the emotion that caused them to eat. Unfortunately, no matter how much they eat, the food won't satisfy their urge; instead, it will make them feel worse when they realize they have consumed so much in such little time.

Most emotional eaters are usually repentant after consuming outrageous amounts of food. They become so ashamed of their eating habits. Emotional eating is not only dangerous to health; it is also frustrating. You probably understand how frustrating it is because you are reading this book to help you curb the habit. Before reading this book, you must have tried to control your eating and failed miserably. There is no shame in that; at least you have recognized the fact that eating like that is a problem, one you need to overcome as soon as possible. That is the first step in your journey to recover and end your food addiction.

And by now, if you haven't established the mindset that eating according to your emotional whims is a problem, you have a lot of mental questioning to do in the nearest future. Determined to cater to needs of all, this book will help you recognize if you are an emotional eater, help you figure out why you do it, highlight the effects of it on your health (both mentally and physically), explain the impacts of it on your social life, and guide you on how to overcome the urges with the right mindset and level of control.

Are you an emotional eater?
Like it was mentioned earlier, identifying yourself as an emotional eater is the first step in the journey to recovery. If you have not identified yourself as one, the questions below will help you out. Try to answer the questions truthfully, you have nothing to gain by lying to yourself.

Do you eat larger portions of food when you are stressed out?
Maybe you had an extremely long day at work, and after showering (or not), you decide to eat a large pack of chips to reward yourself for the day while waiting for your favorite pizza to be delivered. Subconsciously, you already consumed a lot of calories by eating the potato chips, but because you are eating emotionally, you don't consider it as food; rather, it is a snack you are using to reward yourself for the strenuous day you had. And eventually, when the pizza is delivered, you consume it voraciously because you assume you are still starving from the kind of day you had. If you have ever experienced this, answer the question above as "Yes."

Do you keep eating even though you are not hungry, or know you are full?
This question might confuse you a bit, and you may end up answering this question as "False." Before you do that, imagine this little scenario. You are not physically hungry, but you find yourself

opening the refrigerator to find something to eat. You pick out comfort food from the fridge, maybe ice cream, chips, or even a drink, not because you are hungry but just because you feel the urge to eat. Subconsciously, you went to the fridge and started eating based on impulse. If this scenario seems familiar, and it has happened to you recently, answer this question as "Yes." More than 90% of the people reading this book will answer this question as "Yes."

Do you eat because you want to feel better?
Maybe you are anxious or bored, and you chose to eat as an activity to take your mind away from the way you are feeling. A popular scenario that explains this question best is the ice cream break up remedy. Imagine your romantic relationship just ended painfully, and you don't want to eat at all. You just want to curl up in your blanket and cry. After crying for a while, you are done with the crying phase, and you're finally ready to eat but definitely not interested in anything healthy. If you find yourself wrapped up in your blanket watching a sad romantic movie while eating exorbitant amounts of ice cream and chips, you are an emotional eater. A lot of females resort to ice cream after a break up to make them feel better about themselves. Some do feel better but end up regretting that they ate so much. If this scenario applies to you, answer the question as "Yes."

Do you view food as a reward for accomplishments?

A scenario that explains this perfectly was given at the beginning of the chapter. Let's go back to the top shot lawyer and her relationship with food. If she chose to reward herself with a pint of ice cream for attaining such a prestigious position in her firm, she is an emotional eater. If you associate food with accomplishments or any other emotional event, the chances that you are eating emotionally is pretty high.

Does eating food make you feel safe?

Associating food with safety makes you eat when you are under pressure. Once you start using food as a sort of relaxant, you are in danger of eating more than you should in situations that make you anxious or scared. When eating makes you feel safe, you start to think of food as your friend. In some cases, you even have a particular friend you want to eat in a particular situation. Like when you are sad, ice cream is your go-to-friend, chips are your friend when you are anxious, and pizza is for celebrations. If this is how you relate to food, you are definitely an emotional eater. Even if the other questions don't apply to you, once your answer to this question is yes, you are a hundred percent associating your emotions with the food you eat.

Food Addiction

Food addiction and emotional eating can be placed in the same category because they both make their sufferers eat excessively. However, being addicted to food is quite different from eating emotionally. Food addiction is the uncontrollable consumption of a particular food. Food addicts find themselves unable to stop eating a particular food because they have grown dependent on it and are uncomfortable when they do not satisfy their urge to eat the food.

It is easy to confuse food addiction with emotional eating; some emotional eaters think they are addicts, but they are not. Food addiction is like an extreme case of emotional eating; the distinction is not so clear, which is why the similarities and the differences between both cases would be discussed.

Food Addiction vs. Emotional Eating

Similarities

Food addiction is quite different from emotional eating; however, they have one major thing in common; they both make their sufferers consume exorbitant amounts of food. In a way, emotional eating is a form of food addiction. The urges emotional eaters get due to their emotions make them consume junk, and, in some cases, they are fixated on particular junk food. The moment an emotional eater becomes fixated on a particular food, he or she is gradually becoming a food addict.

Differences

The same area of the brain affected by nicotine and other addiction inducing substances is affected when a food addict consumes the food(s) causing the addiction.

When a food addict consumes certain foods (mostly junk foods), a signal is sent to the brain to release dopamine. Dopamine is a chemical present in the brain that is used in the transportation of information between neurons. The neurotransmitter (dopamine) performs many functions; one of them includes the regulation of emotional responses. As soon as the body experiences a pleasurable situation/ emotion, dopamine is released. Examples of activities that could induce the production of dopamine in the body include sex, inhalation or consumption of a stimulant, consumption of certain types of foods (mostly processed foods), smoking, and other forms of stimulating activities.

Under normal circumstances, the release of dopamine is not a bad thing; it's the brain's natural response to pleasure. The main issue with dopamine is the enormous amount of dopamine released after consuming processed junk foods.

After a person consumes a medium-size apple, the brain releases a small amount of dopamine as a reward for consuming a fuel necessary for his or her survival. The brain is wired to release various amounts of dopamine depending on the type or level of pleasure derived from the activity. The problem with this reward system is that most processed foods contain chemicals that induce the production of large amounts of dopamine. A high level of dopamine in the body is not normal, so in a bid to recover the normal levels of dopamine, the brain will desensitize some of its dopamine receptors. With the receptors gone, the individual will need to consume similar or larger amounts of junks to feel such a high level of pleasure. And since there are fewer dopamine receptors in the brain, the dopamine released from healthy or whole foods like apple and orange does not count anymore as your brain will release normal low levels of dopamine, but you won't feel it because you are already accustomed to higher levels of rewards (dopamine). This is why the person involved won't be satisfied with the healthy consumption of apple and will seek out the pleasures derived from eating comfort foods like chocolate and ice cream.

There are two stages of food addiction, the tolerance stage, and the withdrawal stage. The tolerance stages involve the consumption of foods that makes the brain accustomed to high levels of dopamine. The more you eat in this stage, the more desensitized your brain receptors get. The brain experiences withdrawal when a poor dopamine producer like apple does not satisfy the 'fix' as it doesn't reach the level of dopamine it has tolerated. From there, the cravings persuade you to remember and consume that particular food that gave you so much pleasure. The circumstances above also apply to drug and alcohol addiction; the process is the same.

Back to the differences, food addicts consume certain foods because they appreciate the pleasure certain foods give them, they don't associate food with a particular emotion as emotional eaters do. Food addicts eat to get high, to feel pleasure, not because they are bored, lonely, or they want to celebrate.

However, emotional eaters have unknowingly tapped into this knowledge because they know just the food to eat when they want to feel better. Most emotional eaters eat ice cream or chocolate as a cure for sadness, and both of them are known to release high levels of dopamine, which will alleviate their mood. The major difference here is that emotional eaters are eating food to satisfy their emotions while food addicts are consuming food because they crave for it and are already addicted to the 'high' it gives them. Food addicts don't want to experience a particular emotion before they eat; they just want to consume it whenever.

How to identify if you're an emotional eater or food addict
There is a very 'thin' line between both situations. Answering the following questions will help ascertain which one you are.

Do you feel powerless when you're eating?
That moment when you feel like you can't control yourself and you have to keep eating that food, not because you want to but because you have to. An addict consciously eats the food they eat to satisfy their cravings. Emotional eaters do not eat the food they eat consciously; they do it to relieve their emotions. Most times, they don't even realize how much they've eaten until they are stuffed, or the food is finished. This is not the case for food addicts, they eat their food consciously (full knowledge of the amount of food they are consuming), but they don't feel powerful enough to stop.

As you can see, both circumstances involve control, conscious control for food addiction, and subconscious control for emotional eating.

Do you justify or make excuses for your eating?

When you experience cravings to eat junks, do you justify or find a reason to do it? Yes, cravings are really bad and lead a lot of people into making bad diet choices, but they are very controllable. A food addict does not try to control the cravings, they know that eating like that is not healthy for them, but they keep doing it because they can't control the crave and end up making up excuses that allow them to eat the food, in some cases, the excuses are "emotions." If you're eating because of emotions you can't control, you're simply an emotional eater, but if you're conjuring up emotions just so you can eat, you're a food addict. Does that explain the thin line that exists between both cases?

Whether it is food addiction or emotional eating, if your answers to the questions here and earlier in the chapter are positive, you clearly have a problem with food. Now that you have ascertained that your relationship with food is problematic, head on to the next chapter, which will help you define what a normal relationship with food should be.

Chapter Two

Why Do We Eat?

The major reason for eating should be to survive; eating is primal. Apart from that, there are numerous other reasons why people eat. Some people eat because of their culture, traditions, societal expectations, and many more. Some people eat because they are attracted by the appearance, smell, and taste of a particular food. People that eat because of their attraction to the food do it to on compulsion and to satisfy their curiosity. As established in the previous chapter, some other people eat to satisfy their emotions and cravings.

The main reason why a normal healthy human being eats should not be to satisfy a craving but to satisfy their hunger and their need to consume food to carry out their day-to-day activities. However, this is seldom the reason why people eat. Over the years, centuries, and millenniums, the reason why people eat has changed gradually. In the days when men lived in caves and clothed themselves with pieces of fur, food meant survival to them. Nothing else mattered as long as they had food, water, and shelter. They knew the consequences of starvation and did not eat recklessly when they didn't have to.

After men advanced from living in caves to living in actual houses, they developed a steady timetable for eating and called the meal times- breakfast, lunch, and dinner. After a while, they added snacks to the menu. Even with the abundance of food, there was nothing like food addiction or emotional eating because they were stuck to their timetable and rarely ate off schedule. Any deflection from the timetable usually resulted in a missed meal. Our predecessors did not associate food with pleasure or emotions; they just ate because they needed to. The snacks they ate were healthy and did not have any of the side effects modern snacks has on our health.

In the modern world, most people have abandoned the regular food schedule and eat anytime they are able to. Due to their busy jobs and daily activities, they rarely get the opportunity to exercise and burn all the excess calories they consumed. Following the trend of the era, a lot of people started developing problems with food. The problems ranged from anorexia to food addiction, emotional eating, and many more.

Judging from the fact that you are reading this book, you must have one of the problems listed above. Worry not, help is on the way. To help you understand the reason why eating is necessary, I will highlight the basic reasons why food should be consumed.

Reasons for Eating
The very first reason why any man eats is to survive.

There are three basic requirements that every human being living on earth must acquire to live a normal life. They are – food, water, and shelter. Shelter to protect them against the dangers of the world, water to sustain them, and food to give them the energy to carry out their daily activities. The body can go at most twenty-one days without food, as long as the water is consumed regularly during the period. However, even though the person is still alive, he will be a shell of his previous self as he won't be able to carry out his normal day-to-day activities. The weakness that will ensure the starvation process will start in the second week, the hallucinations will start in the third/fourth week, and by the end of the fifth week, the individual's organs will start to deteriorate rapidly. Starvation has a lot of dangerous side effects; some of them are:

Low blood pressure

Reduced heart rate

Numbness

Dizziness

Hallucinations

Faintness

Abdominal pain

Shutdown of organs

Heart attack

Haphazard body temperature

Thyroid malfunction

PTSD

Reduced potassium levels

Abdominal pain, and many more.

The side effects will keep increasing until the individual dies. Therefore, food and water are necessary to ensure the survival of man on earth.

To function at peak level

Apart from eating to survive, you also have to eat enough food to carry out your daily activities the best way you can. If you consume just enough to survive, your body won't perform at its peak level. You won't have the ability to carry heavy items for long, trek long distances, or participate in any activity that requires endurance. Your activity level will be proportional to the amount of food you are consuming. However, this should not be an excuse to overeat and consume unnecessary amounts of food. Eating the appropriate amount of food will make you energized and strong, while overeating will leave you heavy and useless. You will read more about the consequences of overeating later on in the book.

For growth and development

Eating healthy foods that contain the right balance of nutrients encourages your body to develop and grow optimally. Lack of nourishment will result in stunted growth or body defects that may take years to cure. The ideal diet plan should contain all the seven classes of food in the right ration. If two or more classes of food are missing from a diet, the individual consuming the food would be deficient of some vital nutrients needed for the optimal growth of the body.

The Seven Classes of Food

    Carbohydrates,

    Protein,

    Fats and oil

    Vitamins,

    Minerals,

    Roughages, and

    Water.

Each class of food contributes to different proportions of nutrients needed by the body. The type of nutrients required by the body can be grouped into two classes

Macronutrients

Micronutrients

Macronutrients are the classes of foods that are required by the body in large amounts. The classes of food that are categorized as macronutrients are protein, carbohydrates, water, fats and oil, and fibers. When consumed, the macronutrients are converted to energy, which can either be measured in Joules or kilo Calories.

Different classes of food provide different levels of energy. Carbohydrates and proteins produce at least 17 kilo-joules per gram, while fats and oil produce the most with 37 kilo-joules per gram.

Micronutrients are classes of foods that are required in minimal amounts by the body. Examples of food groups that fall into this category are vitamins and minerals. While vitamins and minerals help to nourish the body, it is not required in large proportions. A small amount is able to do all that is needed in the body.

Classes of Food/Food Groups

Protein

The hype protein receives in the workout and dieting community is well deserved. None of the other food groups perform as much function as it does. Every single cell in the body contains proteins. If you consider the level of organization of living things which states that all tissues are made up of a collection of cells and all organs are made from an aggregation of tissues, you will understand that every cell containing protein means that protein occupies a significant percentage of the human body. The percentage was calculated to be around 16%, depending on the weight, size, and diet of the individual.

Therefore, it's a good thing that protein performs a lot of functions in the body. Some of the basic functions it performs in the body are

Due to the fact that most of the tissues, muscles, and organs are made up of protein, consumption of protein can aid the repair of damaged parts in the body. Hence, it is popularly known as the building block of the body.

Protein helps to maintain the regular growth process of the body.

Proteinous enzymes help in the breakdown and digestion of food.

Some protein elements in the body help to transport materials around the body. Materials like blood and fluids in the body.

The immune system is made of proteinous components that help to defend the body against diseases and microbial attack.

Food deposits stored for future use are kept in the form of protein, e.g., Albumin.

As you can see, the effect of protein on health is unmatched by any other group of food. Note that the body, however, does not rely on protein for fuel unless it is absolutely necessary.

The protein structure is made of multiple amino acids, both essential and non-essential. On its own, the body can manufacture some important amino acids for its activities; these amino acids are called non-essential amino acids, while the amino acids that cannot be synthesized by the body are called essential amino acids. Essential amino acids can only be obtained from food. Examples of essential amino acids include arginine, leucine, phenylalanine, tryptophan, and six others. Examples of non-essential amino acids include glutamine, glycine, glutamic acid, and six others. Together, there are 20 amino acids.

Sources of protein

    Eggs

    Meat

    Fish

    Beans

    Almonds

    Oats

    Milk

    Cheese

    Yogurt

    Broccoli

Quinoa

Lentils

Brussel sprouts

The amount of protein that should be consumed in a day depends on the age, weight, and activity level of the individual.

Carbohydrates

Do not be fooled by the low carb diet craze gaining popularity in the past few years. Carbohydrate is good for the body. While protein repairs and grows the tissues in the body, carbohydrate produces the main fuel that is necessary for the running of the body. Your daily diet should contain about 45-65% of carbohydrates, for it is to be a balanced meal.

Everyone's trying to lose weight and have named carbohydrates the bad guy. There are unaware of the important functions carbohydrate performs in the body.

It provides the body with energy to perform activities.

It regulates the level of glucose in the blood

It facilitates the breakdown of fatty acid and prevents the occurrence of ketosis after a long day without eating

Protein generates energy directly in joules, while carbohydrate relies on the phosphorylation of a phosphoryl group before it can generate energy. Sources of carbohydrate include

Oats

Potatoes

Yam

Butternut squash

Rice

Pasta

Quinoa

Couscous

Lentils

Chickpeas

Kidney beans

White bread

Bagels

Banana

Blueberries

Kiwis

Honey, and many more.

You will notice that some of the foods mentioned above were also mentioned under protein; the reason is that no particular food is a hundred percent protein, carbohydrate, or any other type of food group. E.g., honey is 82% carbohydrate and 18% some other group of food. 82% is a really high number, and most of the foods listed above are less than 60% carbohydrate. You must be wondering why they were listed as carbohydrates if they still contain large amounts of other substances, this is because the largest and most significant portion of it was carbohydrate.

Fats

Consumption of dietary fats is absolutely necessary for the regular functioning of the body system. The word "fat" has been associated with a lot of negativity; it's an insult, it's an image, and it's the root of most cases of depression among overweight teenagers. However, while most people would love to avoid anything that has to do with both the word and the food, it plays a major role in the transportation and storage of important materials in the body.

It's a popular misconception that eating fats makes you fat. This is not completely true. Yes, fats deliver twice the energy protein, and carbohydrate food generates, but this won't make you fat; eating foods with high proportions of fats and carbohydrates will make you fat. The results of studies carried out on a group of women who ate foods high in fats, and low in carbohydrate showed that "fat" doesn't make you fat as the women that were observed loss weight instead of gaining weight.

Importance of fats in the body
- Provision of energy

- Part of the structural components of cells in the body

- Carrier of fat-soluble vitamins to the necessary parts of the body.

- The brain is made up of 60% fats.

- Omega-3 fatty acids have been known to perform a lot of healthy actions in the body. Some of them are

- Reduction of blood pressure and prevention of heart-related diseases

One of the three known types of Omega-3, EHA, is used to treat deeper and anxiety.

DHA, another type of Omega-3, is a structural component of the retina in the eye, and low levels of DHA may result in vision problems.

DHA is also known to boost the brain activity of infants and helps to prevent brain defects in infants.

Consumption of Omega-3 supplements helps people with metabolic syndrome manage their condition

Omega-3 helps to fight inflammation, which can result in a heart disease

Autoimmune diseases can be treated with Omega-3

Mental disorders like schizophrenia and bipolar disorders have been managed with Omega-3 supplements.

Omega-3 has been observed to reduce the chances of having certain types of cancer

Omega-3 lowers the risk of developing asthma in both adults and children.

Omega-3, a fatty acid, is known to reduce the level of fat present in the liver and prevent inflammation problems in the liver.

The bones and joints are not left out as Omega-3 is used to treat arthritis and boost the level of calcium in the bones, improving bone strength.

Studies have shown that Omega -3 supplements are more effective in treating dysmenorrhea than ibuprofen.

DHA is known to improve the quality and length of sleep.

Consumption of DHA, a structural component of the skin, helps to keep the skin supple, moist, and wrinkle-free. EPA also helps to prevent premature aging of the skin, prevents the formation of aches and helps with the hydration of the skin.

As you can see, a diet that involves the consumption of Omega-3 at least thrive a week definitely has its benefits.

Sources of Fats

Avocados

Dark chocolate

Fatty fish like mackerel, salmon, and herrings.

Whole eggs

Cheese

Nuts – groundnuts, peanuts, almonds, walnuts, etc.

Chia seeds.

Extra Virgin Olive oil, coconut oil

Full fat yogurt

Coconuts, and many more.

Vitamins

Though required in small quantities by the body, vitamins perform a whole lot of functions. And it is required in small quantities because large amounts of it do more damage than good. A good balance of vitamins among the other groups of food is sure to boost the health of the consumer immensely.

Every single second, the body breathes, it's carrying out activities that require oxygen and nutrients. The performance of those activities gradually deplete the store of resources in the body, consumption of vitamins help to replace them. Failing to consume the small quantity required is sure to lead to a deficiency disease. Some popular vitamin deficiency diseases include

- Scurvy – vitamin C
- Night blindness – vitamin A
- Rickets – vitamin D
- Weak bones – vitamin D, vitamin K

It's almost impossible to list all the functions of vitamins in the body, but it's possible to list the vitamins in existence. They are

Vitamin A (Retinoids) – Fat-Soluble Vitamin

Sources – bell pepper, carrots, potatoes, eggs, beef, peaches, cantaloupe, squash, pumpkin, etc.

Vitamin B1 (Thiamine) – Water Soluble Vitamin

Sources – asparagus, navy beans, Brussels, tuna, spinach, lentils, tomatoes, peas, lettuce, mushrooms, etc.

Vitamin B2 (Riboflavin) – Water Soluble Vitamin

Sources – almonds, eggs, liver, spinach, mushrooms, tempeh, mackerel, yogurt, etc.

Vitamin B3 (Niacin) – Water Soluble Vitamin

Sources – asparagus, corn, peanuts, sweet potatoes, lentils, turnips, salmon, barley, mushrooms, etc.

Vitamin B5 (Pantothenic acid) – Water Soluble Vitamin

Sources – sunflower seeds, liver, strawberries, eggs, mushrooms, cauliflower, squash, etc.

Vitamin B6 (Pyridoxine) – Water Soluble Vitamin

Sources – sunflower seeds, liver, banana, tomatoes, mushrooms, brown rice, squash, etc.

Vitamin B9 (Folic acid) – Water Soluble Vitamin

Sources – papaya, banana, tomatoes, mushrooms, brown rice, squash, etc.

Vitamin B12 (Cobalamin) – Water Soluble Vitamin

Sources – eggs, salmon, trout, cereals, etc.

Vitamin C (Ascorbic acid) – Water Soluble Vitamin

Sources – Bell pepper, guava, broccoli, kale, lemon, pineapple, tomatoes, parsley, strawberries, grapefruit, oranges, etc.

Vitamin D (Calciferol) – Fat-Soluble Vitamins

Sources – sunlight, salmon, mushrooms, eggs, tuna, etc.

Vitamin E (Tocopherol) – Fat-Soluble Vitamins

Sources – sunflower seeds, strawberries, avocado, nuts, green vegetables, olives, etc.

Vitamin H (Biotin) – Water Soluble Vitamin

Sources – banana, salmon, papaya, cauliflower, eggs, etc.

Vitamin K – Fat Soluble Vitamins

Sources – asparagus, carrots, green peas, parsley, green vegetables, etc.

The other classes of food are also equally important; minerals, fiber, and water are basics of a standard diet. However, they won't be discussed in this book.

Physical Hunger vs. Emotional Hunger

Physical hunger is experienced when the body requires sustenance to continue its daily activities. Physical hunger is very different from emotional hunger; it is only experienced when your stomach is empty, and the body needs more energy. It does not prompt you to eat when you don't need to eat, nor does it make you eat excessively. When you are physically hungry, it does not have anything to do with what you are feeling at that very moment; it just means that you're famished, and you need to consume fuel (food) to continue your activities.

The standard meal times are breakfast, lunch, and dinner. Most people experience physical hunger early in the morning (breakfast) and late in the day (dinner). Hunger is felt early in the morning because the food consumed at dinner was used by the body overnight. You may not know this, but the body carries out activities while you are at sleep. Your body replaces worn-out cells overnights, repairs weak cells, and performs a lot of activities that cannot be carried out while you are active. These overnight activities will obtain their energy from the food you consumed before you sleep, this is why you wake up hungry even though you consumed a full meal as dinner shortly before you slept. But the reason for experiencing physical hunger late in the day depends on the activities you carried out during the day. If you did not do anything that requires a lot of energy, you might not even feel the need to eat because you still have some fuel left form the meal you consumed in the morning. However, if you had a stressful day and carried out a lot of strenuous activities, your body will demand that you replace the energy you utilized by sending signals to your brain to remind you to eat. If you try to ignore the signals, your hunger will worsen, and the loss of fuel (energy) will start to show in your body.

Physical hunger has a lot of physical effects, unlike emotional hunger. After a few hours of ignoring the signals triggered by your hunger, you will start to feel the effect of the hunger. Some of the effects include

Dizziness

Nausea

Abdominal pain

Salivation

Lack of concentration

Weakness

Exhaustion

Drowsiness

Shivers

How does the brain signal physical hunger?

The hypothalamus in the brain is responsible for creating the hunger sensation. Nerve cells in the hypothalamus create the hunger sensation by producing two proteins – neuropeptide Y (NPY) and agouti-related peptide (AGRP), which stimulates the appetite of the host.

According to Isaac Newton, for every action, there is an equal and opposite reaction. The same law applies here because when the nerve cells in the hypothalamus produce the hunger simulating protein, nerve cells around the hypothalamus produce proteins that perform the exact opposite function of NPY and AGRP. The proteins produced by the nerve cells around the hypothalamus are called melanocyte-stimulating hormone (αMSH) and cocaine and amphetamine-regulated transcript (CART). αMSH and CART are proteins that inhibit the hunger sensation produced by NPY and AGRP. Whether you feel hunger or not is dependent on the balance and actions of these four proteins.

What controls the actions of these proteins? Hormones circulating in the blood are responsible for maintaining the balance. Ghrelin, a blood-circulating hormone synthesized in the stomach, is known to be the major cause of physical hunger. The stomach increases the production of Ghrelin as it starts to empty and decreases production when it is filled up. When Ghrelin is present in high levels, it will travel to the hypothalamus in the brain and induce the production of NPY and AGRP while inhibiting the production of αMSH and CART. As the stomach fills up and Ghrelin reduces, the blood-circulating hormone will not be able to induce the proteins that cause hunger.

Cholecystokinin (CCK) is another blood circulating hormone associated with hunger. When the stomach starts to get full, it starts to produce Cholecystokinin (CCK) in the small bowel. When active, the hormone is known to stop people from eating more.

Another hormone that stops people from eating is Leptin. It is an appetite-suppressing hormone synthesized in fat cells. The hormone tries to induce weight loss by suppressing the appetite of the individual involved. Leptin production is proportional to the production of fat cells; therefore, people with high amounts of fat cells have Leptin in high numbers.

How do you know if you're physically hungry or emotionally hungry?

The two types of hunger are totally different, and they manifest themselves in different ways.

Signs that signal physical hunger

Growling or rumbling of the stomach.

When the stomach is empty, the noises produced by the stomach become more prominent. The stomach can grumble at any time, but most times, the sound is muffled by the contents of the stomach. The grumbling originates from the muscular activity the stomach performs to mix and transport food from the stomach to the small intestines. In the absence of food, the squeezing of the walls makes the individual experiencing it uncomfortable, and coupled with the noise the stomach makes; he is sure to understand that his stomach is demanding for food.

Lack of concentration

This occurs when the individual tries to ignore all the signals sent by the brain. The brain then tries to get attention by making the individual lose focus on the activity he or she is performing. For a while, the individual may be able to focus, but eventually, the brains always win as it will start generating distractions thoughts about food or some random activity different from the one being performed. It's best to give in at that point because the brain won't give up till you eat, and you won't be able to focus and do anything else.

Weakness

The rumbling/growling of the stomach is followed by a lack of concentration, after which the individual involved begins to feel weak. If the individual is unable to satisfy the hunger at that moment, his or her performance level will drastically reduce as he or she won't have the energy. The body is weak because it needs sustenance (fuel) obtained from food to continue its normal activities. It's not advisable to get to this point before eating; try to eat once your stomach starts rumbling, and you start to feel empty.

Dizziness

After weakness comes dizziness. Some people feel light-headed when hungry; this is because of the depleted glucose levels in the blood, a condition called hypoglycemia. To stop the dizziness, the individual needs to consume a drink or food high in sugar content that can immediately restore the glucose levels back to normal. The reason for experiencing dizziness while hungry is that the body already converted the glucose present in the body to energy to carry out both external and internal activities of the individual. Though not everyone experiences this symptom, it depends on the individual's level of hunger. Some even have it worse and start seeing black spots along with the dizziness. Once it gets to that point, the individual needs to address his or her hunger immediately to prevent further complications.

Abdominal pain

For people with ulcers, waiting this long to eat will only end in pain. Ulcers are wounds on the walls of the intestine, and staying hungry for a long time will aggravate the pain. The stomach produces acid to digest the food consumed, and if there is no food to work on, it begins to work on the walls of the stomach, i.e., the wounds. It is advisable for ulcer patients to eat a snack every two hours, aside from the standard three meals consumed.

If you didn't experience any of these symptoms, and you want to know if you're hungry, ask yourself the following questions:

How hungry am I on a scale of 1-10?
Hunger levels above four need to be attended to with either a snack or a full meal. You do not have to get to a ten before you consume your next meal.

When did you have your last meal?
The maximum time acceptable is five hours. If your last meal was consumed beyond that, you need to find something to eat as soon as possible. It's not all physical hunger that comes with symptoms; some may go unnoticed till you start to experience dizziness. To prevent sudden problems, track the time you eat and eat as at when due.

How to differentiate emotional eating triggers from physical hunger.
Most of the time, it is difficult to know if you are actually eating because you're hungry or because you're looking for an activity to do to take your mind off your present emotion. Bored people are known to consume foods that they do not need to eat, but because they do not want to be bored, they took an interest in food, especially junk food. There are a few tests or questions you can answer to establish if you're hungry or if you just want to eat to take your mind off things.

What do I want to eat right now, an apple, ice cream, or waffles?
If you choose to take the ice cream, you are not hungry, you just want to snack, and it may also stem from emotional hunger that

only the ice cream can satisfy. If you're truly hungry, you'll choose an option that is healthier and more filling like apple or waffles.

What am I feeling right now?

Try to identify your emotions at that moment, if you are able to, you will know whether you want to eat because of how you're feeling or if you are eating because you need to hunger).

Examine your mind and your body

Sometimes it's possible to know if you are hungry by pressing the lower part of your belly. If your stomach feels full, you are not hungry, but if you feel empty after pressing your stomach, it's hunger.

Conclusion

This chapter talked about the reason why human beings eat, the importance of the food to their wellbeing, the types/groups of foods known to man. It also talked about physical hunger and how to differentiate it from emotional hunger.

Chapters one and two defined emotional eating and how to separate it from other type types of hunger. The rest of the book will discuss the impacts of emotional eating and highlight proven methods that will stop you from continuing the habit.

Chapter Three

Emotional Eating and Well-being

Why would eating harm you? There is hardly any gathering or event in life where food does not have a part to play. Apart from the fact that food is as essential as air to us, it plays other roles in our lives. However, this is dependent on your current state of mind. Eating does not always bring about or portray positivity; it can lead to negativity. This is where emotional eating comes to play. Emotional eating establishes a causal relationship between your feelings or emotional state and food. Emotional eating is a consequence of either a positive feeling or a negative feeling.

People eat to reward themselves for a job well done or to comfort themselves when life throws a curve. Quite a number of emotional eating patterns could be linked to childhood habits, which were never passed over in adulthood. For instance, cookies, ice cream, chocolate, etc., may have been used when you were little to reward you for performing a particular chore exceptionally, for completing your homework quickly and accurately, or to comfort you when you were sad or stressed. Emotional eating is a habit that should not be handled lightly. This is due to the fact that emotional eating proves perilous to both your physical and psychological wellbeing. This may be attributed to the fact that emotional eating is not a result of feeling physical hunger pangs, but rather an effort to fill an emotional chasm. Normal physical hunger can be satisfied to a great extent with lasting effects by food; however, hunger due to emotional turmoil or stress is not easily satisfied. Stuffing your face with junk food and other comfort food yields temporary relief from the emotional stress and would not solve your problem. As a matter of fact, it compounds it by making you feel bad about yourself. Hence, emotional eating brings forth negative feelings such as; guilt, queasiness, and the likes.

It is very crucial to be aware of the biggest and the most exiguous negative consequences of emotional eating as the risks cannot be overemphasized. Moreover, if emotional eating is done occasionally and with discipline, it might not necessarily pose a problem. However, if it is indulged too often and without discipline and is tending towards food addiction as you learned in the previous chapter, then dire consequences ensue. Some of them include:

Guilt: On the norm, guilt is not a phenomenon that comes up as a consequence of eating. However, when you eat for reasons other than appeasing physical hunger and gaining the necessary nutritional value, you start to feel guilty. Different personalities feel guilty for overeating or indulging in emotional eating for various reasons. Some feel guilty because they have to hide from friends and family to indulge others because it is just plain wrong for them to, and they know it. Because of the emotional stress the guilt presents, there is potential for more emotional eating, which then leads to more guilt, shame, and, consequently, low self-esteem. If this endless loop of emotional turmoil keeps on, it pilfers your chance at a healthy life experience.

Food addiction: Food addiction is the sequel to emotional eating. When emotional eating goes unchecked, it transcends into excessive eating or overeating and, consequently, food addiction.

Weight gain: Quite a number of emotional eaters indulge in high carbohydrate, high cholesterol, and high sugar content foods to fulfill their emotional hunger. These foods make them feel good, albeit temporarily; however, consumption of these foods without an increase in physical activities leads to a considerable increase in weight, which may or may not lead to obesity. Nobody likes to feel uncomfortable in his or her own skin, which is what this unplanned weight gain will amount to. This awkward feeling further causes self-esteem issues, physical incompetence, confidence issues, and ultimately depression, especially to people who hate being fat.

Obesity: Obesity doesn't just happen. It happens, as a result, the combination of various factors such as; lineage, environmental factors, personal habits, and the likes. A person is deemed obese when his or her Body Mass Index (BMI) is at least 30. Obesity is a consequence of emotional eating, food addiction, and consumption of large globs of high-calorie food without a corresponding increase in physical activities or exercise to burn it. It is crucial to note also that the relationship between obesity and emotional eating is a two-way thing. Emotional eating causes obesity, and obesity causes emotional eating. Obese people tend to spiral into depression, shame, self-hate, and the likes, which produce high negative emotions. These people then indulge in comfort food, which is mostly high in calories to curb and overcome these emotions; hence, emotional eating. Obesity results in both physical and psychological consequences. The physical consequence hinges on health complications such as; Hypertension, Heart disease, Type 2 diabetes, stroke, some types of cancer, digestive problems, and the likes. These health complications are applicable to both men and women. However, obesity also causes problems in the reproductive system in women. On the psychological spectrum, obesity leads to depression and low self-esteem. All in all, these series of events produce a kind of vicious cycle that goes on and on if not checked.

Other phenomena that exhibit one relationship or the other with emotional eating and food addiction, no matter how exiguous are as follows:

Self-esteem: Most likely, you already know what self-esteem means. Notwithstanding, let's talk about it, but with special attention to how it connects to emotional eating. Self-esteem simply means to believe in you. It believes in your capabilities and is very well aware of your strengths and weaknesses. Factors like genetics, life experiences, personalities, social situations influence your self-esteem to be high or low, as the case may be. However, we will focus more on low self-esteem, how it triggers emotional eating, and how emotional eating triggers it.

Low self-esteem encompasses having negative feelings about yourself. Feelings like; I'm ugly, I'm too fat, I'm not smart enough, and the likes. As a result, these feelings make you vulnerable so that you take other people's opinions to heart a little too much. You belittle yourself, and in so doing, you are exposed to emotional turmoil, anxiety, frustration, and depression. To tackle this negativity and to feel better about yourself, you resort to eating the so-called comfort food even when you are physically full and do not need it. Eating then becomes a defense mechanism against these feelings, hence, emotional eating.

On the other side of the coin, emotional eating results in low self-esteem, how? One of the consequences of emotional eating previously mentioned is guilt. The guilt from overindulging, from eating when you are not supposed to make you feel shame and regret. Then you start doubting yourself, your resolve, feeling bad about yourself. All these culminate in reduced self-esteem and confidence. These play out in a vicious cycle until steps are taken to mitigate it.

Depression: Depression is a grave mental disease that influences your thinking, your feelings, and your actions. A depressed person is like a changed person. He loses interest in things that used to excite him, he is always fatigued, he changes his eating habit by eating more than normal or eating way less than normal, he doesn't feel like himself which develops into low self-esteem and thought of death and suicide become the other of the day. The status quo of depression is loss of appetite and subsequent loss of weight.

However, its association with obesity and emotional eating results in the manifestation of a special type of depression, which is depicted by an increase in appetite and, subsequently, a gain in weight. Based on this, depression can be denoted as a bi-directional phenomenon that is a trigger for emotional eating and also a consequence of it.

Furthermore, it is important to note that there exists a chain reaction among depression, emotional eating, and obesity. Feelings of depression trigger emotional eating in most people, which then may or may not lead to obesity, depending on some factors already previously stated. On the other hand, an emotional eater has the tendency to fall into depression as a result of weight gain from the indiscriminate consumption of palatable foods (foods high in sugar and fat).

Emotional eating, depression, and obesity all culminate in various serious health complications that are very dire to your way of life and overall wellbeing.

Health complications: Health complications such as high blood pressure, diabetes, constant fatigue, and stroke are the order of the day for emotional eaters. The magnitude of health complications you may experience is dependent on your health history and body system makeup. Suppose there is a long history of high blood pressure or diabetes in your family, then, it means you have a higher susceptibility to these health complications compared to someone with no history of the diseases. Therefore, as an emotional eater, the higher cholesterol, high sugar food you consume, the more health complications you are susceptible to and vice versa. The most common and mostly unavoidable health problems that may arise are as follows:

- Hypertension
- Diabetes
- Osteoporosis
- Cardiovascular disease
- Chronic fatigue
- Stroke
- Infertility in women

Emotional eating could birth eating disorders

Eating a little bit more than usual to commemorate a happy occasion or a festival is normal, especially if it happens once in a while. However, when this becomes too often, and the effect starts to pile up, then it is not good. Eating driven by emotions leads to eating disorders. Let's expatiate on some of the most common ones.

Binge Eating Disorder

Binge eating disorder denotes a lack of control in eating, eating at inappropriate places, and at inappropriate times, eating till you are uncomfortably full and eating till you start feeling guilty from it and disgusted with yourself. It is a psychological ailment that occurs mostly among overweight and obese people. Binge eating is a type of food addiction defined by addictive overeating. It is triggered by anxiety, boredom, stress, and depression. Binging is not easy to diagnose as a lot of people hide it. The diagnostic process includes; physical exam, a study of family health history, and eating behavior. For further diagnostic purposes, binging at least twice a week within three months followed almost immediately with extreme guilt and shame, confirms you are afflicted with this emotional disease. This condition can last for many years with serious health problems (infertility issues in women, obesity, and the health problems associated with it) if left untreated.

Anorexia Nervosa

People who are obsessed with their weight are usually the sufferers of Anorexia or are at risk of getting it. They eat very little quantity of food and exercise a little too much to keep their weight down. Even when they are at the right weight or even underweight, they believe they are overweight. They do everything possible to lose weight, to the extent that their health begins to deteriorate, and their body image starts to get distorted.

Both men, and especially women, are susceptible to this disorder. This may be attributed to the belief that thinness denotes high self-esteem; thus, it is not all about food. Some of the symptoms of anorexia include:

Frequent refusal to eat

    Very frequent visits to the gym

    Insomnia

Use of medicine and the likes to induce purging or vomiting

Dehydration

Social withdrawal

Low blood pressure

Frequent feeling of fatigue

What triggers anorexia in people?

Perfectionist tendencies and obsessive-compulsive personalities. With this trait and leanings, they are never satisfied with their weight and body shape.

Social pressure is also a very common trigger, especially amongst teenagers and young adults of the female variety. Thinness is what is in vogue and most fashionable these days.

Genetics. The genetic makeup of certain people puts them at a higher risk of anorexia.

What are the consequences of Anorexia?

Muscle loss

Osteoporosis

Deficiency in vital nutrients essential for optimum growth

Irregularities in the menstrual cycle for females

The decrease in testosterone in males

Anemia

Bulimia Nervosa

Bulimia Nervosa, also known as bulimia, encompasses the characteristics of binge eating disorder and all its consequences. Bulimia is one of the most debilitating eating disorders that can potentially kill the sufferer. Bulimia is denoted by the consumption of a bizarrely large quantity of food within a short time span. This act is then followed almost immediately by an attempt to circumvent weight gain by purging what was ingested from the body.

It is important to note that purging does not only involve vomiting or use of laxatives, herbs and diuretics and other medication, enema, regular fasting, and excessive exercise after eating.

Bulimia is triggered by an intense fear of weight gain, anxiety disorders, boredom, intense dieting, stress, and depression. It is not easy to diagnose as a lot of people hide binging and purging efforts. The diagnostic process includes; physical exam, the study of medical history, and eating patterns. Bulimia can afflict anyone regardless of gender, social, and economic status or age, with consequences of serious health problems that still linger even after recovery from the disorder.

Intense binging tears the walls of the stomach, causing stomach acid to sip into the rest of the body.

Erosion of the enamel of the teeth, tooth decay, and gum disease due to repeated vomits.

Heart disease, arrhythmia, and heart palpitations; the heart cannot withstand constant vomiting; hence, the heart issues.

Infertility issues in women.

The critical difference between binge eating and bulimia is that:

> Binge eating = compulsive overeating without purging.
>
> Bulimia = compulsive overeating plus purging effort to lose the weight gained.

Who Are the People Susceptible To Emotional Eating?

Everybody has a tendency to indulge in emotional eating. Negative feelings or trauma are not restricted to just a group of people. Everyone feels bad, sad, anxious, shock, shame, and the likes occasionally or at least once in a while. This fact cannot be disputed; it is a fact of life. However, the rate at which different personalities feel differs and is dependent also on the magnitude of the trauma or problems being experienced. For instance, there are some situations in life such as; loss of a spouse, an injury, or humiliating experience, which may seem bearable for you to some extent but may cause someone else to shut down physically and emotionally complete.

Emotional eating is a response to strong emotions, both positive and negative. In simpler words, your emotions have the tendency to trigger emotional eating. The kind and quantity now eaten depend on you and your circumstance.

Emotional eating as a coping mechanism may have been developed or adopted right from childhood into adulthood, for some people. For some, it starts at the adolescent stage, while for some others, an event or series of events triggers emotional eating at adulthood. Let us discuss the factors that trigger emotional eating in people at various stages in life.

Emotional Eating in Children

The category of children who take solace in food and snacks when feeling unhappy or indulge in sweets and the likes when happy did not inherit this behavior. They most likely picked up this habit from their parents/guardian, the home environment, and the community at large.

In general, children's susceptibility to emotional eating is dependent on the strategies the parents employ to deal with their children's emotional situation, especially during the important formative years their behaviors begin to advance. Parents who use food to soothe and reward their kids as the case may be, increases the risk of their kids becoming emotional eaters in their teenage and even adult years. The normal reaction to emotional distress is to eat less because stomachic activity decreases, thereby suppressing physical hunger when there is emotional hunger. Despite this fact, children tend to emotionally eat more rather than eat less as they come of age.

The method of giving children food to quench emotional hunger even when they are not physically hungry, not only triggers emotional eating it also exposes them to other eating disorders such as binge eating disorder, anorexia nervosa, and bulimia nervosa disorders.

Emotional Eating in Adolescents

What do teenagers worry about? They worry about relationships, body image, popularity, Grade point average (GPA), and so on. All these issues culminate in emotional distress, which is managed in various ways. It is at this juncture that the type of parenting influences how they react to emotional angst.

In a situation where a child has learned to suppress emotional hunger with food, such a child will not be able to normally deal with emotional distress without the involvement of one comfort food or the other when they mature into teenagers and then adults.

Apart from parental psychological influence, teenagers tend to be swayed by what is trending. They tend to copy what their peers are doing. Therefore, the risk of teenagers becoming emotional eaters also rests on external influence. Simply put, because teenager A ate a whole bucket of ice cream when she got an F in algebra, teenager B also decides to do the same because it looks "cool" in the process discarding the normal route when dealing with dejection or a setback. This method might actually stick, thereby converting teenager B into an emotional eater. When the consequences start to pile up in the form of weight gain, guilt after indulging, teenager B starts to find ways to reverse the effects. This further results in more eating disorders, especially bulimia nervosa.

Emotional Eating in Adults

Emotional eating in adults can occur through various channels. Some adults have been brought up to use food as a coping mechanism right from childhood and have not dropped it or cannot. Some adopt the practice of emotional eating as a result of trauma, stress, or emotional distress that occurred when they were already adults. However, women are more emotional eaters than men. This fact can be greatly attributed to the natural emotional makeup of women in general. Everyone has their own share of problems and things that stresses them. They also have ways they cope that don't involve emotional eating. Using food to cope is actually easy, even if it is just a stopgap fix 90% of the time. Hence, we are all prone to emotional eating and subsequently affiliated eating disorders.

This chapter focused on the demerits and dangers associated with emotional eating. There are always two sides to a coin. Emotional eating is not so bad, after all. As we have negative emotions, we also have positive emotions. The responses to these emotions as regards food should also be positive. In the scheme of things, food as a coping mechanism is much more acceptable to other negative and debilitating health ones such as; drugs, excessive alcohol, and even dieting. Frankly speaking, it is irrational and impossible to completely eradicate emotional eating based on only its dangers and demerits. Food brings people together, food is a very crucial piece in the fabric of every history, food is culture, food is traditional, and food is used to portray love. The makeup of every human comprises the emotional aspect and the logical aspect. These two parts work together to create a balance, which is how emotional eating can bring about a positive impact on our wellbeing.

Chapter Four

What is Emotion?

To the layman, emotion is what you feel. Not just feelings by merely physically touching the skin, but feelings generated from chemical reactions in the brain as a result of the information generated by the sense organs (eyes, ears, tongue, nose, skin). Based on common knowledge, emotion is regarded as a synonym of feelings. This consensus is untrue as emotions and feelings have different meanings, although they are dependent on each other. Emotions are generated subconsciously while feelings are generated consciously such that without emotion, feelings cannot be generated.

There exist several definitions of emotion, with each one trying to capture what emotion really means expediently. However, emotion is a multifaceted phenomenon that cannot be captured in a single fell swoop. Therefore, emotion could not possibly be classified under one umbrella of mental states. It is rather a phenomenon comprising of different mental responses that change to fit different mental experiences. For instance, the classification of emotions into positive and negative emotions cannot stand because there are some situations where the so-called negative emotions portray positivity. For example, the feeling of hate for evil people or evil things, and the feeling of anger towards injustice. These two examples relate to positive outcomes from the so-called negative emotions. Therefore, emotion is ingrained with a multifariousness of quality, intensity, and direction.

The Roles of Emotion

In other to understand the purpose of emotions in our lives, we need first to be conversant with its components; the subjective component, the physiological component, and the behavioral component.

The Subjective Component

The word subjective indicates an action completely taken within the mind. Emotions come from within the mind; hence, they are subjective. People do not often experience emotions in their unadulterated forms. For instance, if two people witness an event that induces anger, one of them might just be mildly annoyed while the other enraged. They both feel anger but at different intensities. Furthermore, feeling two emotions at the same time simultaneously is also a lot common. For example, feeling happy and nervous on your wedding day.

The Physiological Component

Emotions manifest at times, physically. For example, hand tremors from anxiety, knee jerk for a surprise, and heart-racing from fear, etc. These physical responses reveal the physiological component of emotions and are coordinated by the autonomic nervous system, which is in charge of the involuntary response to stimuli. There are two (2) categories of changes in the body as a result of emotion; external changes, and internal changes.

External changes

These are visible and observable changes that enable the identification of emotion in the body, sweating, changes in body language such as a chin lift, muscle rigidity, knee jerk, etc., change in facial expression and changes in the volume and texture of the voice, goosebumps, etc.

Internal changes

These changes are as a result of the stimulation of the Autonomous Nervous System (ANS). The ANS comprises of the sympathetic and the parasympathetic divisions. The sympathetic division gets the body ready for fight or flight by stimulating the adrenal gland to produce adrenaline during emergency situations. The adrenaline travels round the body, causing the following internal changes when the vital organs are stimulated; pupil dilation, increased heart rate, increased respiration rate, reduced saliva secretion, changes in brain wave frequency, etc. The parasympathetic division, on the other hand, restores the energy expended to express emotion.

The Behavioral Component

This component is all about the true projection of emotion. For instance, a smile to indicate happiness and a frown to indicate annoyance, which is pretty general emotional expressions. People from different cultures express emotions in different forms and at different times. This is where emotional intelligence (the ability to correctly recognize emotional expressions) comes to play.

The functions of emotion are:

Emotions Influence thought processes

Unlike computers, human memories are stored with the emotions felt at the time the memories were made. For this reason, we recall happy memories faster when we feel happy and angry memories when we feel angry. Emotions also influence our thought processes. It gives meaning and impact on our values, attitudes, and even our speech. Emotions also aid critical thinking, depending on the intensity of the emotion. Intense emotions might just make it a tad bit difficult.

Emotions help us understand each other better

Our emotional gesticulations and facial expressions give other people clues about what you are thinking. Emotions are tools of communication that have been in use since the beginning of time. Emotions facilitate the formation of bonds with family and friends. True emotions, when projected, enable our loved ones to know what we are actually feeling and not what we tell them.

Emotions facilitate decision-making

What we feel about a certain person or event determines the action we will be taken regarding it. Emotions also help us to make decisions every day, even decisions as simple as what to eat for breakfast or what color of cloth to wear to work. Emotions show us in certain situations what is trustworthy and what is not. These emotions might have been generated through sight or smell or even human gut feelings. In some other situations, our emotions act as a light in the dark.

Classification of Emotion

Humans are complex, so why not their emotions? There are so many related and differentiated emotions that trying to single them out into separate entities is like pouring water into the ocean. In that case, where one emotion begins, and the other ends will be hard to establish. Despite this fact, a lot of psychologists have tried to classify emotions notwithstanding the tendency of humans to experience different emotions at once, thereby adding a layer of complexity. Despite the added layer of complexity, we must understand our emotions because they inform our judgment, decisions, and actions.

Therefore, emotions can be broadly classified into basic emotions and complex emotions. Basic emotions are the bedrock of all other refined emotions. They are the foundation from which all other emotions are deducted. Bearing in mind the variety of thoughts we express; it is no wonder they can get the better of us. There are so many phrases to describe the emotions that emerge in life, but all feelings are derivations of five core emotions; happiness, sadness, shame, fear, and anger. Complex emotions are more particular and eugenically specific than basic emotions. Here, we will be focusing on the basic emotions since they are the foundation.

Happiness

Happiness is one of the most desirable emotions known to man. It is characterized by feelings of joy, contentment, satisfaction, gratification, and wellbeing. Despite the fact that happiness is one of the most desirable emotions, different people and cultures derive happiness from different situations and events. Happiness is a very personalized emotion such that what makes you happy might not make the other person happy and vice versa.

When you are happy, it doesn't only reflect in your disposition; it also reflects on your physiological and psychological health. On the other side of the coin, unhappiness has been associated with feelings of loneliness, depression, anxiety, stress, and deficiency in the state of health.

Happiness is usually expressed physiologically, through a smile, a relaxed body posture, and a pleasant voice.

Sadness

Sadness is also a basic emotion. It is characterized by feelings of sorrow, distress, grief, depression, and the likes. The intensity of this emotion varies depending on the person and the cause. A situation might occur that results in a mild upset for someone but deep dejection for someone else.

When you are sad, it doesn't only reflect in your disposition; it also reflects on your physiological and psychological health. Sadness is usually expressed physiologically through crying, quietness, slouching body posture, and a depressing tone of voice.

Fear

Fear is a vital emotion for survival. Once you face some kind of danger and you get spooked, this message is sent to your brain, which activates the sympathetic nervous system, also known as the fight or flight response to stimuli. Your muscles tighten up, your heartbeat accelerates, and you become short of breath. All this physiological reaction increases your alertness, priming your body to either run or take a stand.

Just like every other emotion, not everybody experiences fear alike. A situation that triggers fear in one person might not result in another person. When we feel the danger in our immediate surroundings, the way we respond to it is identical to the way we respond to anticipated danger, which we tend to think about as anxiety typically.

In some cases, people search out fear-inducing activities in the form of extreme sports. They appear to thrive and even get pleasure from it. However, repeated exposure to those kinds of scenarios will result in familiarity and acclimatization, which might scale back emotions of fear and anxiety. This is often the thought behind the desensitization procedure, which gradually decreases sensitivity to fear.

Fear is usually expressed physiologically through dilation of the pupils, accelerated respiration and heartbeat, tremors, etc.

Anger

Anger is characterized by feelings of annoyance, agitation, hostility, and frustration towards others. Like fear, anger also activates the sympathetic nervous system, also known as the fight or flight response, once a threat generates feelings of anger. While anger is usually thought of as a negative feeling, it may just be an honest response to a provocation. It may be used to portray your stand in a relationship or a situation.

Anger may become a retardant, once it's excessive or expressed violently or in ways, which are harmful to others. Furthermore, anger may result in mental and physical consequences. Unbridled anger has been associated with coronary heart diseases, alcohol consumption, smoking, aggressive driving, and other health risks.

Anger is usually expressed physiologically through sweating, frowning, red cornea, ear-splitting voice volume, etc.

Shame

Shame is the emotion that surfaces when you feel disappointed or has negative feelings about yourself. Shame has the potential to alter the way we see ourselves and may result in long personal and social difficulties. Although shame is completely individualistic, shame is completely different from guilt and embarrassment. Guilt is sometimes understood to involve negative feelings regarding an act one has committed, whereas embarrassment deals with a social group reaction. Shame, on the opposite hand, involves negative feelings regarding oneself, which may be relived publicly or privately.

Chemical Composition of Emotions

An overview of the nervous system

A series of processes are involved in the generation of emotions. Emotions are generated through the arousal of the nervous system. The nervous system is a complex system generally comprising of the Central Nervous System (CNS) and the Peripheral Nervous System (PNS). These two parts of the nervous system work together take in sensory input, process the information collected, and then release the corresponding output.

The CNS is made up of the brain and the spinal cord, which is located inside the skull and the vertebrae. The bones protect the CNS. The PNS, on the other hand, is made up of nerves that run to and from the CNS. The nerves, unlike the brain and spinal cord, are not encased in protective bones; they are scattered throughout the body. Based on the functions of the nervous system, it can be divided into the Somatic Nervous System (SNS) responsible for voluntary actions by connecting the CNS to the organs and skeletal muscles, and the Autonomic Nervous System (ANS) responsible for involuntary actions such as our heartbeat, sweating, pupil dilation, digestion, etc. The ANS is further categorized into the Sympathetic Nervous System, which activates in emergency situations, and the Parasympathetic Nervous System, which activates when the body is in a relaxed state. The ANS, the limbic system (for example, the amygdale responsible for fear), and the hypothalamus are the aspects of the nervous system predominantly involved in the physiological aspects of emotion.

There are a lot of disparate emotions which includes but is not limited to; happiness, elation, excitement, joy, exuberance, enthusiasm, passion, sorrow, remorse, sadness, mortification, guilt, embarrassment, bashfulness, regret, pity, terror, petrify, afraid, panic, shock, apprehension, insecurity, uneasiness, fear, frantic, intimidated, caution, nervousness, anxiety, worry, fury, rage, outrage, enrage, mad, upset, annoyed, irritation, frustration, agitation, depression, agony, disgust, touchy, dejected, hurt, misery, melancholy, cheerfulness, gratitude, relief, satisfaction, glad, contentment, shame, pleasant, tender, pleased, mellow, distress, jealousy, loathing, surprise, remorse, zest, trust, hysteria, euphoria, anger, hatred, indifference, pride, pleasure, displeasure, confidence, grief, zest, hostility, apathy, awe, boredom, affection, angst, contempt, courage, curiosity, etc.

A very significant amount of chemical reactions occur in the brain within a given time span. Chemical reactions take place due to synapses through which neurons transmit messages making use of neurotransmitters (example, adrenaline). The neurotransmitters that help the body function properly and also help to establish a balance are as follows:

Dopamine

As you learned in chapter one, dopamine is regarded as the reward hormone. This organic chemical is characterized by dual functionality. It serves as a neurotransmitter and a hormone. It is pivotal to our survival and fine living. Dopamine is released by the kidneys and the brain with several pathways. Dopamine does not make us feel good; rather, it motivates us to indulge in things that give us pleasure. When dopamine is released into the pleasure center (an area just below the thalamus), pleasure is felt. The brain always recalls what triggered the pleasure previously felt as it creates a dopamine pathway for it so that when the event is repeated, the pleasure widens the dopamine path already in the brain. Irregularities in the dopamine levels are the major cause of the majority of the nervous system diseases such as; Parkinson's disease, psychosis, schizophrenia.

Serotonin

Serotonin is also known as the happiness hormone. It generates feelings of a serene mode of happiness. Serotonin is responsible for emotions such as arousal, aggression, and mood. It is produced in the brainstem and released against disquiet and vasoconstriction. Deficiencies in serotonin levels result in depression, anxiety disorders, compulsive behavior, aggressiveness, low self-esteem, and impulsiveness.

Endorphins

Endorphins are neurotransmitters produced in response to the stimuli of pain or stress. Endorphins are produced in the central nervous system and pituitary gland. When we undergo strenuous exercise, endorphin production is triggered. In fact, all activities that bring pleasure, such as eating, sex, music, etc. facilitate the release of endorphins. It is important to note that it is easy to get addicted to endorphins because of the euphoric feeling it generates. The deficiency of endorphins results in mood swings and extreme contrasting emotions.

Oxytocin

Oxytocin, an organic chemical, is produced in and released by the hypothalamus and pituitary gland, respectively. Close contact with people facilitates the release of oxytocin. It is also known as the love hormone, which is released during and after childbirth. Oxytocin is responsible for romantic love. It creates bonds and inhibits the part of the brain that is associated with fear and anxiety. Deficiency in oxytocin culminates in depression, fear and anxiety, and poor communication.

Estrogen

Estrogen is regarded as the reproduction hormone. It can be found in both men and women; however, its quantity is insignificant in men as it is majorly a female hormone. Estrogen is produced in the endocrine system and is released into the bloodstream. It is in charge of female reproduction, puberty, menstrual cycle, and maintaining the level of cholesterol. Estrogen works with other hormones such as serotonin and endorphins, by boosting their levels in order to facilitate the emotion of the feel-good kind. There are three types of Estrogen in women: Estrone, Estradiol, Estriol, and Esterol. Each of these is produced at different stages in a woman's life span.

Estrone is released during menopause.

Estradiol is released when women become of age to start giving birth. It is mostly found in the ovaries.

Estriol is produced majorly in the placenta and is released during pregnancy.

Esterol is also produced during pregnancy.

Balance is very important when it comes to hormones in the body. It shouldn't be low or high but at the right level. When Estrogen is low in the body, feelings of anxiety, depression, and mood swings occur. On the other hand, if it is too high, it leads to constipation, acne, and cancer of the breasts in the extreme case. Apart from the fact that it is a naturally produced hormone in the body, it is used in the form of medication as contraceptives, menopausal hormone therapy, etc.

Progesterone

Progesterone is produced in the corpus luteum located in the ovaries. Progesterone is in charge of regulating the process of ovulation. It plays a vital role during the menstrual cycle. Progesterone works hand in hand with Estrogen to achieve emotional balance in the female reproduction arena. While Estrogen facilitates excitement, progesterone facilitates relaxation and calmness. Irregularities in progesterone levels result in anxiety, irregular menstrual cycle, headache, and mood swings, among others.

Testosterone

Testosterone is regarded as the reproduction hormone in men. It can be found in both men and women; however, its quantity is insignificant in women as it is majorly a male hormone. However, some women have it at slightly higher levels than normal. This the reason why some women grow beards and mustache, which is primarily a male thing. Testosterone is produced in the testes and is released into the bloodstream. It is in charge of male reproduction, puberty, libido, muscle strength, and bone mass, among others. Testosterone works with other hormones such as serotonin and endorphins, by boosting their levels in order to facilitate emotion. When Testosterone level is too high in the body, it increases aggressiveness, impulsive behavior, anger, mood swings, and an exiguous amount of empathy. On the other hand, if it is too low, it leads to anxiety, insecurity, and a reduction in self-confidence, depression, among others. Apart from the fact that it is a naturally produced hormone in the body, it is used as a medication to treat low testosterone, transgender hormone therapy, cancer of the breast in women, bodybuilding, and so on.

Adrenaline

Adrenaline, also is known as epinephrine, is the fighter hormone. It serves a dual purpose of hormone and medication. It is produced in the adrenal gland and in the medulla oblongata by neurons. It is released into the muscles and bloodstream in response to involuntary stimuli such as blood pressure, pupil dilation, and respiration, among others. It is majorly released during emergency situations where the body is perceived to be in danger. That is, it is triggered by emotions like fear, startle reaction, and the likes. Too low levels of epinephrine cause depression, while too high levels of it can cause mental diseases like schizophrenia. Adrenaline is administered as medication directly into the muscle by the use of injection to treat health conditions such as cardiac arrest, asthma when other treatments fall through, allergic reactions, etc.

Acetylcholine

Acetylcholine is an organic chemical messenger located in the autonomous nervous system. It is released by the neurons to stimulate the muscles, enhance concentration and memory. It exhibits an inverse relationship with serotonin such that as one increases, the other decreases. It stimulates the brain and facilitates the release of some other hormones like dopamine and serotonin. It also regulates emotions like fear, anger, rage, and aggression.

Cortisol

Cortisol is produced in the adrenal gland. It is a coping hormone. It helps the body to manage stress levels, so it doesn't overwhelm the body system. When a lot of it is released, it leads to anxiety, hypertension. On the other hand, if it is too low, it leads to emotional eating and some other eating disorders, alcoholism.

GABA

It is a chemical messenger produced from glutamic acid. It is responsible for inhibiting excitement in the brain. It serves as a natural emotion tranquilizer, reducing fear anxiety and panic. Low GABA levels in the body are associated with the bipolar disorder condition.

Chapter Five

Eating and Emotional Intelligence

How to Identify and Express Your Emotions Properly

Identifying our emotions hinges a lot on emotional intelligence which also hinges on four major skills:

Self-perception

Self-control

Social perception

Relationship control

The relationship between our lives, us, and our emotions is the relationship between a ship, passengers, and the captain. In this analogy, we are the passengers; our life is the ship while the captain denotes our emotions. The captain is the boss and frankly speaking the most important participant because he is the controller, the driver who helps us to sail the ship in the best possible and beneficial direction. Therefore, the importance of emotions in our lives cannot be overemphasized. We need them to survive, to make decisions, to take actions, and to communicate.

We need to be able to identify our emotions to understand them. We are complex creatures, and so are our emotions. Therefore, it requires a lot of skills and effort to recognize and understand our emotions. It would have been marvelous to have started this journey since childhood, as we would have had years to work at it. Notwithstanding, it is better late than never.

Now that we have acquiesced to learning, identifying, and understanding our emotions, the next on the agenda is to hone the four emotional intelligence skills. To do that, we need to dissect each skill one after the other. But first…

What is emotional intelligence?
This is the ability to identify command and express emotions in all situations in other to achieve success personally, professionally, and socially. When the sense organs pick up information or a sensation, it enters the brain at the base near the spinal cord then travels to the frontal lobe where logical thinking takes place. However, it passes through the limbic system where emotion is produced on its way to the frontal lobe. This indicates emotion works on the sensation before it is reasoned out. This link is the physical origin of emotional intelligence, also known as emotional quotient (EQ). Emotional intelligence demands efficient communication between the areas of the brain in charge of reason and emotion. Emotional intelligence is vital in other to succeed. Almost every event that occurs in our life extracts an emotional response, whether we are aware of it or not. We are complex entities; therefore, we need to be

ready to make an effort to understand our corresponding complex emotions.

Self-Perception Skills

Self-perception is not about rooting out your secrets. It is your ability to correctly discern your own emotions and knowing what rocks your boat. To go about these, you need to painstakingly think about what you are feeling at a time, the origin of the feeling, and what triggered it. Self-perception skill is the foundation of achieving emotional intelligence. If you have self-perception down pat, you will be able to carry out analysis – identification of strengths, weaknesses, and opportunities before diving into any venture or when confronted with a foreign or even familiar situation.

Strategies

The following are strategies to help you make optimum use of your self-perception to effectuate positivity in your life.

Stop attaching labels to your emotions. As humans, we always want to categorize things into neat little boxes. We tend to do this for emotions too, such that we categorized some emotions bad and some good. We then try to avoid feeling or get rid of the so-called bad ones. Do not avoid an emotion because you don't like it, or it makes you uncomfortable. If you do, the opportunity to learn and grow your emotional quotient will also be lost. Hence, when you get overcome by any emotion whatsoever, let it run its course because if you don't and begin second-guessing, it distorts the actual message of the emotion. This hinders the self-perception process.

Observe the immediate effect of your emotions on people close to you; you will be surprised by how much your emotions affect those around you, especially those in close vicinity when your emotions were outpouring. Having the thoughts that your emotions are yours and yours alone will not allow you to decode it effectively. Therefore, take the time to reflect on your emotional expressions, ask those in your immediate surroundings how it made them feel. This will give you the tools to decide the type of effect you want to affect.

Objectify your emotions; when you feel, it manifests physically at least 80% of the time through increased heartbeat, loss of breath, hand tremors, etc. Therefore, in other to understand your emotions, take the time to read the physical changes that occur when you feel. As they say, practice makes perfect, so carry out simulations of emotions so as to repeatedly read the physical responses that occur. This way, you become an authority in discerning your emotions physically, even before you are aware of it mentally.

Comprehend what makes you tick; having the knowledge of whom and what makes you go off is very critical in your self-perception journey. It makes it or them less daunting. Investigate those persons or situations that violently trigger your emotions. Take notes.

Record your daily events, so you don't get overwhelmed. Record the emotion, what prompted it, and how you reacted. It is a good strategy to adopt as it makes available references for future consultations.

Question your actions. Emotions catch you unaware, so don't just let it be. Look for the source, ruminate on the reason you acted the way you did. The more you study your actions, the more control over your emotions you garner, and the more unlikely your emotions take you unawares.

Do not lose sight of your **principles**. If your self-perception journey is all about understanding your emotions so as to make decisions you can live with, therefore losing sight of your values is out of the question. If you have to write your values somewhere then read it every morning when you wake up, please do so.

Not everyone can recognize patterns or take cues or even run simulations. For this reason, critically observe the emotions of characters in movies, books, and even the lyrics of a song, especially the ones that reflect your own emotions. You can learn a lot about your own emotions from it.

Seek unbiased opinions. Emotions are subjective since they originate from the mind, although they can be seen through physiological reactions. There is a tendency of there being a biased account of your emotions since you are the examiner and the examinee. This is why the employment of external opinion would not hurt but rather authenticate the information you get.

Self-Control Skills

Self-control provides you with the tools to wade through oceans of uncertainty and come out at the other side relatively unscathed. Flexibility is a key factor for effective self-control. Self-control is impossible without the proper perception of your emotions. Successful self-control is dependent on your ability to adjust and adapt in situations that do not conform to the status quo.

Strategies

Now that you know what makes you tick emotional-wise, the following are strategies on how to harness the skills acquired to manage your emotions such that, you are able to choose how you react to your emotions, how to control it, so it doesn't get the better of you regardless of the situation.

Take deep breaths when you feel an emotional explosion coming on. This might look very simple and insignificant, but it is actually very effective in the scheme of things. When you take a deep breath in such that your tummy swells; as a result, your brain is supplied with a lot of oxygen, which will have a calming effect on you. In some situations reacting to an emotional trigger might be a mistake that will prove detrimental to your plans or even your relationship with other people, therefore taking a deep breath gives you time to think again, weigh your options, and at the same time, clear your head.

Publicize your objectives. When you set a goal or aim to achieve something, do not keep all to yourself as it is easy to give up since it is all subjective. Therefore, create a clique of people you always trust to have your back, tell them all about your plans. They will keep asking about your progress; they will keep encouraging you when you hit a snag. In a sense, even if you don't mind failing when things get hard, you will not want to so that you will not disappoint your fans, so to speak.

Do not jump to act; this is all about being patient. When a situation that provokes a reaction occurs, take your time to react, give it a day, two, or even weeks. Take apart the feeling and analyze every facet of it. You will be rewarded for your patience. It is either during the waiting period, something else comes up to nullify the emotion, or you are able to prevent yourself from making decisions that will be next to impossible to take back.

It will not hurt to engage the expertise of those with emotional self-control skills when trying to manage your emotions. Ask them for their opinions; tell them to share their own experiences, the strategies they employed, the hurdles they went through, and how they were able to tackle them. This is the classic learning from the mistakes of others rather than learning from your own mistakes analogy.

Control the conversation with your thoughts; our thoughts speak to us all the time. Research posited that we have an average of fifty thousand thoughts per day, both positive and negative. It is now up to you to decide which of these thoughts you allow to influence your actions. Control your thoughts, or else they control you.

See your success even before you actually succeed; it has been proven that our brains do not only process the information from our physical senses; they also process the ones from our imaginations. For instance, looking at a lion and imagining seeing a lion is perceived as the same by the brain. Therefore, imagine seeing what you want to see, hearing what you want to hear, feeling what you want to feel, and your brain takes the message, processes it, and then produces the corresponding organic chemicals and the projected emotions into your system. So if you imagine positive things, you will feel positive emotions.

Capitalizing on your strengths instead of your flaws allows you to be open-minded and flexible in all situations. Open-mindedness and flexibility are two of the most crucial attributes of an emotionally intelligent person.

The self-perception and self-control skills are all about knowing you, your emotions, your actions, and your triggers. Now, an emotionally intelligent person is not only competent about personal issues but also competent about social issues (his/her relationships with others).

Social Perception

It is not all about you. You need to take into consideration other people's perspectives. To do this, you need to build your listening skills and observation skills. Social perception is the ability to put yourself in others' shoes without letting your own feelings or perspectives influence your judgment. Social perception involves acquiring emotional antennae or sponge capable of picking up what other people are thinking or feeling from their gesticulations, facial expression, and voice tone.

Strategies

The following strategies, if employed, will help you acquire social perception skills.

Listen to what the body has to say; everybody has a language their body speaks. The body speaks through the eyes, the face, the shoulders, the arms, the fingers, the legs, and the feet. It is now left to you to listen. To be able to, you need to learn what any movement made by those body parts mean. For example, when people look you in the eye, their eyes steady when talking, then the deduction is they are trustworthy. Being able to read and interpret body language is a very crucial social perception skill you must acquire to achieve emotional intelligence.

Perfect your timing; it involves asking the right questions, at the perfect time for it, while taking into consideration your object's mood and state of mind. For instance, it is bad timing for you to ask a person who is clearly in a bad mood for a favor.

It is said that, when you prepare and plan your activities properly, you will be able to avert poor performance or failure. This saying teaches us to always prepare before diving into any venture so that you do not get sidetracked when something unexpected happens. If you want to venture into anything, stop and take the time to map out all the details, including possible adjustments for unforeseen circumstances, so that you don't commit blunders as a result of improper planning.

Forget the past for a moment; to be socially aware; you need to be able to let go of the past so that you can harness the full potential of the present. Letting go of the past does not just happen because you put off a switch, you have to make an effort that may sometimes involve mentally dragging yourself from ruminating about the past so as to focus on the present at least for a moment.

Watch movies that help you increase your emotional intelligence; watching movies can serve as practice material for the development of your social perception skills. Therefore, select a movie, play it. Immediately the movie starts, begin the exercise. Study the emotional language of the actors and actresses, take note of how they relate with one another. Pinpoint the body language, the facial expressions, the eye movements, the arm and leg movements, the movement of the fingers and feet, and shoulder movements. Try to interpret what those body cues mean based on the emotional atmosphere and storyline in the movie.

This practice method is fun and at the same time, yields productive results for your emotional intelligence acquisition.

Hey! Don't look at you for a minute; yes, it is difficult just to stop and take the time to observe what is going on around you, the people around you when there are a lot of things to do. However, this is a requirement for social perception. This helps you to deduce what makes people do the things they do and say the things they say.

Try to understand other people's cultures and traditions; this may also help you deduce why people are the way they are. It helps you to be able to treat them how they want to be treated. This also requires long periods of listening, observing, and asking or questions, which are also requirements for social perception.

Relationship Control Skills

Relationship control is the ability to incorporate the combination of your self-perception, self-control, and social perception skills in your interactions and relationships. This gives you the tools you need to be able to see and harness the advantages and see and discard the disadvantages of all your relationships with people. Relationship control does not only helps build relationships, but it also helps you maintain those relationships for as long as you want those relationships.

Strategies

Establish a line of communication; make yourself approachable so that people can get to know you, at the same time, apply your social control skills in getting to know the people around you. Make sure there is an open line of communication between you and your colleagues or your friends or your partner or any other person you deal with at close range at all times. You might have a lot of things in common, which you would not know without showing interest and asking questions. As a result, you are able to forge stronger bonds than you anticipated or hoped.

Clean up your act and put your mouth where your money is communication-wise; the first thing you need to do is to make sure there is no chance for people to be confused about what you really mean. It doesn't cut it if you say something, but your body language says something else. People tend to believe more in what is said than what is heard. To make sure you are not misunderstood, use your self-perception skill to identify your emotions and your self-control skills to choose the ones you want to project and the ones you do not.

The second thing you need to do is to make sure u don not forget to appreciate when it is deserved and to apologize when you are wrong. This will go a long way in solidifying your relationships.

Dictate the time, direction, and magnitude of your emotions; to achieve this fit is a lot of work. It is not easy. For instance, anger, which is one of the basic emotions that creates the groundwork for emotions like fury, rage, etc., is not easily dissuaded or inhibited. However, if time, direction, and magnitude are incorporated into it, there is a possibility of productive outcomes you can use to amplify your relationships. Furthermore, to be able to use anger judiciously, you need to employ your self-perception skills to grade your anger from the most exiguous irritation to the most blinding rage by identifying your triggers. Then you choose the magnitude that conforms to the time and the person it is being directed at so that your relationship will not suffer. This is what relationship control is all about.

Make sure there is synergy between what you want to affect and what you actually affected. It is like when you are trying to say something, but you end up saying something else instead. In order to avoid such occurrences, use your social perception and your self-control skills to appraise the situation on the ground before you speak and act.

The social perception and relationship control skills are all about knowing what makes other people tick, their emotions, their actions, and their triggers so that you can establish productive and lasting relationships with them.

Now that we have established that it takes the skills of emotional intelligence to be able to identify, understand, and express our emotions properly. It is important we also learn how to change already established bad habits, so we can move forward to achieve the best emotional quotient we can.

How to Control and Change Superficial Behaviors

Superficial people scrape the surface of anything and everything. They do not have the wherewithal to deal with serious and demanding situations. They are shallow in their thinking, words, and actions. When a superficial person is confronted with a situation, he or she does not have the wherewithal to deal with it efficiently and thoroughly. Emotionally speaking, superficial behavior is a result of having a ridiculously exiguous measure of emotional quotient. It can be said that a person exhibits superficial behavior due to emotional deficiency.

Superficial behavior can be controlled through the adoption of emotional intelligence skills, self-perception skills, self-control skills, social perception skills, and relationship control skills. Employing all the strategies of attaining these skills, which have already been outlined, will go a long way.

Emotional Regulation

Emotion regulation is the employment of emotional intelligence skills. It is a learned skill as we are not born with it. In order to regulate our emotions, we have to be able to identify, accept, and adapt our emotions optimally based on the situation. Therefore, it requires us to be skillful in self-perception and self-control.

Emotion regulation could be an extremely personalized exercise. Some folks were raised with well-grounded self-management skills as youngsters, whereas others had very little to no behavioral steerage growing up. Still, emotional regulation could be a talent, and like most talents, it is learned and improved with regular training.

Apart from the added obvious advantages, like feeling higher within the immediate term, well-established emotion regulation skills are capable of enhancing your emotional health in the long-run, improving work performance, enriching personal relationships, and even prompts more quality overall health.

Furthermore, emotion regulation helps you through solving your emotional problems by re-identifying them so as to be able to proffer accurate and functional solutions.

Emotion regulation helps to improve your state of mind and reaction style, which will help you to build your emotional intelligence. Moreover, for anyone wanting to boost their regulation skills, it is vital not to feel embarrassed as a result of undesirable or uncomfortable emotions. Everybody has them. It is how you handle them that matters.

Chapter Six

How to Deal with Emotional Eating

As you must know by now, it is the urge you feel that triggers you to eat. When you feel this trigger, rather than turning to the food, you need to find other outlets for your emotions, sometimes you think emotional eating helps you cope with your daily emotional states, but the truth is that it only serves as a temporary source of relief and in the long-run, you will discover that it leads to poor health, weight gain, and other health implications discussed in the earlier chapters.

In this chapter, I will be discussing how to stop emotional eating once you have recognized your trigger.

General Acceptance
It is difficult for most of us to accept some of the traits that we deem negative, while we feel good about those traits that are positive. Unconditional acceptance is the core of loving oneself. This means that even though your body is not perfect, you don't rate yourself as being unworthy. Accepting your body size, shape, and perceived flaws do not mean you would not have preferred to be born with a different body, nor does it imply that you can't improve on yourself. Accepting yourself implies loving yourself unconditionally. It means embracing who you are and the way you

look. People generally think that self-acceptance means resignation and giving in to your mediocrity, but the opposite is the case. When you accept yourself for who you are, you want to get better. Self-criticism, and rejection create a sense of helplessness and hopelessness, which in turn can lead to depression and loneliness, and when this happens, we turn to food to fill in for the emotional hunger we are experiencing. When we accept ourselves, we are not constantly looking for approval from others. When you acknowledge and enjoy your inner environment, you create room for personal growth and transformation.

Accept your feelings

This is another way of acknowledging the truth about your situation like it was said earlier; it does not necessarily mean resignation. When we accept our reality, we broaden our options for tackling a particular problem. When we accept our feelings, we can find a way to respond to them. It also encompasses recognizing your feelings, understanding the cause in a non-judgmental way. For example, "I don't like the way I look," this is just a thought you are having without feeling shame and despair. Accepting a situation is a gradual process; you don't just arrive at it once. Before you can be able to accept your feelings, you must identify it first. You can just find a quiet place where you can be alone and ask yourself how you are feeling. You can begin with, "I feel...." The statement, for example, "I feel worried." Doing this will help identify the emotions you are feeling.

You can put this acceptance into practice; you don't need to start with the most challenging situations of your life. Examples will be given in a series of steps below

My weight is sixty-pound, and I've been steadily gaining weight since the break-up, but I can't stop turning to food when I think about it.

I tense my body by raising my hands in a way that the forearm is at a 90-degree angle to my body, I clench my facial muscles and fist by raising my eyebrows and pursing my lips. I feel uncomfortable, and this break-up seems heavy in my heart.

As I release my body, the tension is being relieved, and I feel ready to move on with my life. I am ready to commit to a plan to move forward.

Accepting involves having the willingness to accept your situation rather than trying to control the reality of what is happening. When we are willing to accept the feelings that come with a situation, then we are ready to accept the situation. Willingness is the persistent practice of acceptance, regardless of whether the outcome is good or bad. There is an important point to note, if we are practicing acceptance and willingness to control how you feel or how to feel less pain, then you are not truly practicing, in this case, you are using willingness and acceptance as an evasive strategy. You also need to find a way to return to acceptance if you move away from acceptance. For example, you can accept that you have to stop using food to cope with your feelings if you want to learn how to manage them. The exercise below is going to help us notice the emotions we are feeling and how to practice acceptance for it.

Exercise

To practice this exercise, pick a situation where you will encounter intense emotion. While in this situation, notice the feelings you are having from a distance without passing judgment. This will help create awareness of all the emotions you feel and how willingly or unwillingly you want to accept these emotions. You can create a scale for your emotions and willingness, also note the tendencies and urges that show up.

Situation: gather all the facts about the situation that leads to these emotions.

For example, I went to a colleague's birthday party at my favorite restaurant, where I overate last week for emotional reasons. I am anxious about repeating the same pattern. I'm still hurt over the recent criticism from my boss.

Thoughts and interpretation – Don't want to dwell on my boss's criticism; it's okay to have an occasional longing to eat emotionally, but this doesn't have to dictate my behavior.

Rate your emotions: you can create a scale of 1- 10, with 10 being the extreme version of the emotions you are feeling. For example

Anxiety- 6, Willingness-9, I felt anxious about overeating and willing to feel anxious

Hurt-7, Willingness-3, I didn't want to feel hurt.

Tendencies and urges: felt the urge to indulge in my favorite blueberry muffin like the last time and complain about my boss's criticism to my friends.

Practice acceptance: observed all my emotions in a non-judgmental way, accepting that it is okay to have them, I practice a technique for relaxing my body when I feel discomfort at not ordering my favorite dessert.

Expressing your Emotions

Binge eaters eat in response to a lot of triggers, but let's talk about how you can express your emotions when you are feeling these triggers rather than turning to food. Sometimes we need to forego these negative emotions that act as our triggers, for the positive ones, do not allow them to overwhelm you too much. There are several ways of dealing with your emotions

- Exercise
- Meditation
- Music
- Exercise

It is a well-established fact that exercise can be used to manage stress. It is one of the major techniques used for stress management. The role of exercise in emotional eating often depends on individuals' motivation. Although the role of exercise on emotional eating has not been established scientifically due to limited research in this area. Apart from stress management, exercise helps increase the rate of our metabolic activities, burn calories, increases the metabolism of fats, and regulates the appetite. Exercising goes beyond fat management, it goes a long way to regulate your mood, most of the time, and this is majorly the cause of emotional eating. Generally, exercising improves the overall quality of life. Exercise can be a moderate or vigorous activity, depending on the level of effort applied to it.

There are various exercises to do when you want to take your mind off stress and anxiety.

Jogging

Running

Walking at a brisk pace

Cycling

Skating

Skiing

Mowing the lawn

Hiking

Fast rope jumping

Fast dancing

You can also perform some resistance exercise and flexibility exercise.

There are times when we give excuses about exercising due to some situations. There are ways you can overcome these excuses and still exercise. Some examples of excuses include:

- **You normally feel drained after every exercise or too tired to exercise**

It may be that your diet is not supporting you i.e., your body is not deriving the needed energy from it. To remedy this, there may be a need for you to boost your hormonal system first. You can also start increasing your daily activities by doing the following

> Taking the stairs instead of the elevators, even if it is just a flight

> Park your car a few blocks away from your workplace and trek the remaining distances

> Dance to your favorite music

> Do some garden work

> Mown your lawn

> Perform gentle exercise.

- **You don't have the time to exercise**

If you don't have the time to exercise, re-evaluate your priorities, and get creative enough to carve some time out. Exercise does not take too much of your time, especially when it can be broken into a 5-10 minutes session. You might decide to go for a walk on your way home from work.

- **Exercise is boring and uncomfortable for you**

When exercise is boring and uncomfortable, it's not compulsory to join a gym; you can just pick something you enjoy doing, it might be a sports activity, dancing swimming. Just pick something you will be comfortable with. If you dislike moving your body in general, concentrate on picking activities that are tolerable for you at first and vary them gradually as you continue. Try and reframe your mind against negative thoughts about exercise with the positive ones.

Exercise doesn't make a difference in your weight

First, are you in the habit of starting and quitting exercise programs? You start exercising and then stop when you feel that you are not losing weight. When you start again, you start with the more vigorous one that will quickly burn you out. This leaves you dejected and unmotivated. You think, "after all, it's not working." You could start with a moderate-intensity activity that raises your heart rate, which can be broken into increasing sessions. For example, your first session is 5 minutes; the next might be 10 minutes. Disprove the notion that this little exercise doesn't count unless it is vigorous. Taking this short exercise reduces the risk of burning out and injury; also, the overall feeling of having completed a session gives you great motivation to do more.

Set realistic goals

When you want to start a session, set realistic exercise goals for yourself. Keep in mind that starting less is better and feels positive about your accomplishment, no matter how little it may be. You can keep track of your activities and progress in a journal or calendar; also, you can write down the benefits of the exercise to your body.

N.B- as much as exercise is good for the body, we should be careful not to overdo it. Over-exercising can result in hormonal imbalance and adrenal exhaustion. Do not ignore your body signal telling you to slow down, below are some general signals to watch out for

Having a problem sleeping

Complete exhaustion soon after exercise or feeling exhausted the following day

Dreading exercise

Experiencing soreness that doesn't heal quickly

Having a frequent need for stimulant such as sugars, caffeine, etc. to keep going

When you are experiencing this, it is a sign that you are over-exercising, and you need to reduce your activities and have quality rest.

Music/sound

Music takes your mind off difficult emotions; you can also listen to the sounds of nature, such as the chirping of birds, gentle breeze. Many people regard listening to music as a soothing activity that helps comfort, organize, or calm us. Music also has a therapeutic effect, remember to pick music that will calm your mood rather than agitate it.

Meditation

Meditation is another way of dealing with stress and expressing our emotions. Meditation helps you to quiet your mind and relax your body. It can be defined as any activity that keeps your attention anchored to the present moment.

Jacobson's relaxation technique

This type of relaxation is common in the western world; it is simple to perform and effective. To perform this technique, there are steps to follow:

The first step in performing this technique is to make yourself comfortable

Take a deep breath, make sure the air from your abdomen is expelled completely (do this five times) imagine those emotions leaving your body with each breath.

For the muscles in the following part of the body listed below, contract the muscles for 10secs and relax them for 20 seconds, while doing this, concentrate your thoughts to the feelings of the relaxation and contraction of these muscles

Abdomen

Back

Shoulders

Thigh

Neck

Back

Feet

Face

Conclude the exercise by taking two deep breaths while directing your thoughts towards the feeling of relaxation in your body.

Mindfulness within reach

Another exercise technique to do is Mindfulness within reach; it is a type of meditation technique that is used to manage and modify emotions making you more aware of things around you. Here are the steps for using this technique

The first step is making yourself comfortable

With eyes closed, sit in an upright position (you might decide to sit cross-legged if this is comfortable for you, or sit upright in a chair)

Take a deep breath and concentrate on your breathing

Pay attention to the sensation you are feeling in your body: if you experienced tension in some parts of your body like face, neck shoulder, try to relax those muscles.

Take note of all the thoughts passing through your mind without passing judgment.

Start observing this for 2min each day, gradually increase the length of time until you get to 10-15 minutes. Some apps can help you to observe this better.

Here are a few tips that will help you incorporate mindfulness into your lifestyle

When you wake up in the morning practice the meditation technique

Observe your posture whenever you sit or stand and note your tension point, and try to stretch.

How to Tolerate Distress

Bad mood often leads to a bad decision; negative moods affect the way we think. Generally, when people experience negative emotions, they tend to involve themselves in risky behaviors as a way of ridding themselves of the negative emotion they are feeling.

For example, when you are experiencing loneliness, you might call an Ex from a bad break-up in a bid to rid yourselves of the loneliness, and if your advance is not reciprocated, you turn to other things as a distraction, e.g., food without thinking about what this behavior will cost you in the long-run.

What is distress tolerance?

Distress tolerance is defined as the ability to accept and farewell with difficult emotions that will lead to pain and that any irrational behavior will lead to more pain. You can develop a strategy to tolerate both physical and emotional pain. If you want to know whether you are struggling with intense emotion, use the following to check

- You numb yourself to intense emotion

- When you have intense feelings, you tend to lose control and act impulsively

- You are in denial when you are feeling painful emotions

- Your feelings overwhelm you

- You can't stop thinking about your problem.

You will notice that the foundational problem is acceptance, in coping with distress, the first step you have to take is accepting the situation before you start taking other steps like noticing emotions and mindfulness. Practicing mindfulness is very important because it helps you notice your emotions, urges, and accept your pain.

Distress tolerance is different from emotion regulation, but both require mindfulness. Emotional regulation applies to ordinary emotions experienced, and it requires coordination, but distress tolerance has to deal with extraordinary overwhelming emotions. When you rate the emotions you are feeling on a scale of 1-10, those emotions higher than 7, there is a need for distress tolerance.

When you are experiencing difficult emotions, and you urgently want to get rid of the pain, you want an instant fix for your intense emotion, something that will take your mind off what you are feeling at that moment, and at the same time, it will be pleasurable. Food often fulfills these criteria; it can both be a source of pleasure and distraction. Relying on food to cope with intense feelings may hinder you from developing other ways to cope with these emotions, and when there is no strategy in place to cope with these emotions, there is no way to break the cycle of emotional eating. We have no control over the way we think or what we feel, but we do have control over what to do about them. Distress tolerance can be applied in the following situations:

Dealing with overwhelming emotions: for instance, you might be angry over a friend's criticism, but you know your friend is right; you can practice distress tolerance to deal with your anger. Try to view the criticism from a neutral point.

Managing feelings that arise in response to behaviors you have engaged in: you can practice distress tolerance when you feel guilty having indulged your cravings for cinnamon after a fight with your father.

Accepting the discomfort or pain that arises from letting go of routine behavior: the discomfort you feel when trying to quit smoking or when you are trying not to finish a whole jar of cookies after taking a bite of one.

We have discussed how to practice mindfulness earlier; note that in practicing these, you will notice the emotions you felt and the direction these emotions take you towards or away from.

Skills needed to tolerate distress

Some specific skills can be used to tolerate distress. Majorly, distress tolerance entails self-soothing and acceptance. This set of skills is the complete synthesis of both soothing and acceptance.

Acceptance

Like it was said earlier in the chapter, it all boils down to acceptance. Acceptance and willingness are the two basic ways of dealing with overwhelming emotions, it is one of the major tools of distress tolerance, as discussed earlier, it is a way of accepting your emotions and coping with what your feelings without having to find other means of distraction, here, we are going to learning additional way of practicing acceptance.

Accepting your food cravings

Accepting your food cravings means not forcefully trying to control any food you encounter. Accepting your food cravings help you to understand that trying to control your food cravings only increases the sensation and awareness about the particular food. In accepting your food cravings, you are not trying to influence any food that crosses our path; you are not actively trying to control your cravings. When we are in crisis, we tend to look for a quick fix, but accepting your cravings in the face of this crisis requires less effort on your part, yet this acceptance is highly beneficial to you.

Accepting hunger

It is not healthy to deprive yourself of regular meals as this will create more problems. But for some people, emotional eating may be due to fear of possible hunger. Emotional eaters view hunger in an all-or-nothing way. Experiencing great discomfort with mild hunger might maintain emotional eating, this remedy requires you to purposely miss a meal to keep track of your discomfort and get rid of your hypothetical fears, but if you are in the middle of a crisis filled with a lot of intense emotion, it is not advisable to skip a meal. And if food is unavailable, you can practice accepting hunger at this point.

Accepting set back

The inability to accept setbacks gives room for more setbacks. Viewing setbacks in the all-or-nothing terms lead to a relapse. For example, if you consider ice-cream as your weakness and you also consider taking a spoon as sinful as taking the whole ice-cream, you are more inclined to finish the whole bowl of ice-cream, you are making it difficult for yourself to accept the tiny setback. Kindly notice the way you make sense of these actions. Notice that a spoon of ice-cream is not the same as the whole bowl. Committing a tiny mistake and then concluding that you are weak may lead to you giving up. If a person who is trying to quit smoking, smokes a cigarette, him concluding that he is weak and out of control from just smoking a cigarette can lead to him smoking the whole pack of cigarette. Accepting that mistakes do occur, accepting your emotions, thoughts, and urges is more beneficial than setting a rigid self-discipline rule.

Soothing

Soothing is one of the basic ways of tolerating distress. The best way to curb impulsive or mood-driven behavior that arises as a result of overwhelming emotions is to practice self-soothing. Having rational thoughts when we are experiencing overwhelming emotions can be a difficult challenge. You can think and plan soothing activities that will lead you in the opposite direction of what you are thinking. Soothing is a bridge between emotions and emotional actions that helps you to deal with your distress without creating more problems. You may soothe yourself by listening to music, immersing yourself in a warm bubble bath with scented oils and candles, plan a trip, etc.

Cost and benefit

If you repeat the same pattern of behavior when faced with intense emotion, you might want to consider writing the cost and benefit of your impulsive behavior's when you are in a calm and rational state of mind. For example, emotional eating might be beneficial in that it creates a pleasurable distraction for you, but the cost of this is extra-calories and short-term distraction from your feelings. You should also indicate whether the effect of both the cost and benefit will be short-termed or long-termed. You can outline the behavior you indulge in when experiencing intense feelings, the cost and benefit of engaging in the said behavior and indicate whether the effect of the behavior is either short term or long term.

Sight

Sight is also another way of dealing with intense emotions. Going to the park, looking at photographs, noticing people moving up and down the street can serve as a distraction from your feelings, just doing this we relax you and take away your concentration on what you are feeling at that particular moment.

Seek the support of a friend or proper channel

Seeking support is very helpful, especially in the time of pain, but not all support act as a buffer against pain, certain support can escalate your stress level. It is up to you to seek the support that will provide a calming effect for you. For example, you can seek support by setting up a meeting with your psychologist, attending group therapy, calling a friend, listening to calming messages, and calling a helpline, as will be treated later in this chapter.

Seeking meaning to life

Seeking meaning in pain facilitates acceptance. Accepting pain as something we experience in the course of living can go a long way in helping us deal with our emotions, i.e., experiencing pain is a normal part of life. All people experience a deep sense of imperfection, but finding meaning in your experience helps you to connect and empathize with others. Seeking meaning requires both the practice of mindfulness and flexible thinking.

The above are tools used in tolerating distress when faced with overwhelming emotions.

Practicing self –compassion
Practicing self-compassion means being open to your pain and suffering. Practicing the feeling of kindness towards oneself, having a non-judgmental attitude towards yourself is a key part of practicing self-compassion. Especially when you are struggling with emotional eating, planning your meal, and eating mindfully. When you occasionally indulge in some emotional eating, you approach it calmly and do not judge yourself harshly. Self-compassion is about honing your skills and effort to comfort yourself. When you judge yourself too harshly without accepting that some of these setbacks occur because you are human only gets you stuck to emotional eating. Having self-compassion protects you against emotional distress and promotes good health. To simplify it, having self-compassion includes

- Noticing what you are thinking and your emotion in a mindful manner

- Accepting that these experiences are part of being human

- Practicing understanding and self-kindness towards oneself

Self-compassion is like practicing acceptance and mindfulness, but in this case, it is directed towards ones' self. Practicing self-compassion shows you that you are bound to face challenges and setbacks, but like every other person, you are not perfect. Practicing self-compassion builds on mindfulness, distress tolerance, and emotional regulation. When you practice self-compassion, you activate your self-soothing system, which is more useful than being stuck with guilt. If eating serves as your way of dealing with negative emotions, self-compassion creates a form of awareness. Compassion reduces the distress you feel, and the guilt associated with binging, and this helps improve your eating. Feeling guilty about indulging yourself leads to more emotional eating. Practicing compassion towards yourself may facilitate your closeness with others, practicing gentleness, compassion towards yourself may help you develop the skill and practice it towards others. Having the ability to understand yourself from non-judging positions helps you to understand others better. This helps in creating a connection with others.

Another big issue is self-criticism, which leaves you vulnerable and dependent on food for comfort. When you are deep in self-critical thoughts, it is hard to notice others. Like it was said earlier, practicing compassion helps. Sometimes when you have indulged in emotional eating, you begin to seek assurance from people by asking them whether you have gained weight or not. When someone passes a harsh judgment on the way you eat or feel, you lash out and then feel anger or guilt, which can trigger your emotional eating all over again. You can practice self-compassion by noticing the urges ask for other people's comments or your own yearning to dwell on other people's comments about your body. Having a high or low expectation of yourself is not very kind, so also is treating yourself indulgently or restrictively. You can modify how you treat yourself. Self-compassion helps you in managing your emotions, connecting with others, and improving on your diet.

Incorporate flexibility into your way of life
When you focus majorly on your weight and diet, you are bound to struggle in the end, so also is focusing on your job, it will affect your social life. What I am trying to say is that you should not focus on just one aspect of your life. Set other priorities for your life, be flexible

Establishing self-connection
Self-connection is when you notice your inner emotions, thoughts, and needs, search for your distress signal and quickly correct them to keep your emotions in a balanced state. Disconnection from one's self is one of the primary causes of emotional eating. When you are disconnected from yourself, you are cut off from your emotions i.e., your basic signals. You still experience negative emotions, but your emotional eating is not only a way to soothe and distract yourself from these emotions, but you also derive pleasure from eating. In this case, you are trying to fill up on something outside yourself. Like I said earlier, accepting your emotions is one of the first steps in determining what you need.

How to Practice Self-Connection

Practicing self-connection starts with an inner conversation. Our self-talk is like having a conversation with ourselves; we all engage in this self-talk, whether we are aware of it or not. We have internal conversations like "I shouldn't have any more cake, but this cake tastes so good; I will just have a little more." These voices are sometimes the voices of a caregiver, a sibling, a parent, or a mentor. These voices represent the thinking part of us; they often influence our decisions. Our thinking self can be a supportive, kind nurturer, a destructive critic, or a neutral voice. These voices are part of our personality. If your inner voice is the supportive and nurturing kind, you can look into yourself for the support and comfort you need without having to turn to other sources. But if your inner voice is the destructive and criticizing one, you are regularly doubting and beating yourself up, feeling unworthy and depressed, you might turn to food for comfort. Disconnecting from your inner voice is a natural way of putting a stop to this harsh, judgmental voice. When you disconnect from your emotions, you lose the opportunity of getting in touch with your authentic feelings. If you don't find the right way to express your emotions properly, they come out in other ways leading to reckless and impulsive behaviors. Unexpressed emotions create havoc on your body, mind, and spirit.

Practicing self-connection is similar to practicing acceptance;

Ask yourself about the way you are feeling at that moment

Ask yourself about what you need to deal with the moment

User your inner compassionate voice to assure and comfort yourself.

Try practicing inner conversation in these situations to assure and comfort yourself

When you want to use food, gambling, alcohol, internet surfing drug as a distraction.

When you are experiencing negative emotions like anger, anxiety, shame, helplessness, fear, loneliness.

When you are bored, unmotivated or disconnected

When you are constantly worried about something or having a lot of judgmental thoughts.

When you are stress and about to turn to food for comfort.

Sometimes when you feel overwhelmed by your emotions, it can be a sign that you have been disconnected from them for a very long time. It shows you have been using food to calm yourself to reduce being overwhelmed by this emotion. It is also a sign that you need to develop your self-soothing skills. When these emotions surface, you may feel vulnerable, anxious, and overwhelmed. You can just take a walk or listen to music to calm yourself. For some people, it is just too overwhelming to allow their emotions to surface; this is common for those who have experienced trauma in the past. When their emotions are about to surface, they quickly find what will soothe and calm them because they have this impending feeling of being out of control, or they are dissociated from themselves or the world. Accessing this feeling can dredge up an unresolved wound that you are not ready to face. You can employ the help of a professional therapist or a nurturing friend to provide support for your feelings and how to move on. When you feel overwhelmed by your emotions, there are ways to stop overreacting and acting out your feelings.

Identifying your emotions: as discussed earlier in this chapter, we have to know what we are feeling.

Let go of other people's pain: When you identify your feeling, asses them whether they are truly your feelings or a reflection of someone else's feelings, for example, that of a parent or caregiver. Sometimes we can be carryon their emotions without even knowing that we are doing it. When you acknowledge this emotion and realize you are responsible for these emotions, you can then be able to stop taking responsibility for it.

Share your feelings with others: expressing your feelings opens doors for connecting with others. It gives room for growth and learning in a relationship. Sharing your feelings can make you feel vulnerable, and if your emotions are not well received, you can feel rejected and hurt, but on the other hand, it helps you feel better. It is important to share your feelings gradually until you are more open and comfortable about sharing them.

Identifying your need: when you have been disconnected from your emotions for such a long time that you don't even have a clue of what you need to deal with it. For example, you don't have any idea of what you need, or you know your needs, but you don't know how to meet them. As an emotional eater, your basic need might have been ignored during your childhood years, leading to us seeking support and encouragement from others. Sometimes this craving to have our needs fulfilled might feel like a physical hunger such that we turn to food, which acts as a temporal and pleasurable fulfillment of our need. After identifying your needs, it is very important also to practice acceptance. It is okay to have these needs; they are fundamental to human nature.

Meeting your needs: After you have identified your needs, you can now be more specific about this need. You ask yourself some basic questions like what it would take to meet your needs, the way it would be like if these needs are met. For instance, you identify the need for love, will I receive more affection? Once a need is identified, it takes flexibility and creativity to meet those needs. Most times, it is easier to identify and meet physical needs than emotional ones. This is the time where we put our thinking self into action. For instance, you identify that you get off on adrenalin and would love to go on an action-filled trip but don't have the time to do so, you can hike an unexplored area. When you have identified ways to fulfill your need, you have to focus on this need with the intention to follow through. Following through is important because makes you achieve your set goals. Take baby steps that allow you to meet your needs, making big plans, and not fulfilling them can make you feel like a failure with the conclusion that you might not be equipped to meet your needs.

Expressing your own need: Expressing your needs is another form of self-care if you feel selfish when you are expressing them, keeping mind that it is no more selfish than exercising or eating healthy food. Making your needs know to others shows you respected them enough to tell them your need instead of expecting them to read your mind. This way, you are acknowledging that you feel worthy enough to ask others. When you have been disconnected from your need for a long time, your first time at expressing them can seem demanding, aggressive, angry, and cold. For example, if you make the statement, "I'm sick and tired of not being taken seriously." Others might be less inclined to consider these needs. Writing down your need in a journal, and practicing the way you will express them to another person can be helpful. For your request to be taken seriously, we need to consider the feelings and needs of others and deliver your request with understanding and kindness. You can make a statement like, "I understand that you are busy, but I will appreciate it if you listen."

Catching and Reframing Self-Defeating Thoughts

Have ever noticed how your thought can quickly change moods. Potentially scary news can create anxious thoughts that are hard to shake. A rejected advance from a romantic interest can lead to agitated thoughts and irritable mood. Research has shown that an average person has about twelve thousand thoughts in a day, which is twelve thousand chances of feeling good or bad. When your thought tends towards the positive and optimistic ones, we feel as if we can conquer the world, but when your thoughts tend towards the negative and unpleasant ones, you feel anxious, depressed and frustrated. This negative and unpleasant feeling can lead to us wanting to find a source of distraction and distraction. There may be a need for you to recycle these self-defeating thoughts. These thoughts can be about anything ranging from your body to what happened in the past. Your thoughts start the moment you open your eyes in the morning, and if these thoughts are negative ones, that is the start of a bad mood. For instance, Clara is awake, and the first thing she thought about is how the day is filled with so many activities and how she will never be able to get through it. How she hates her job and should have quit it a long time ago. She catches her reflection in the mirror, oops! Here comes another self-criticism, "I look so fat, my skin looks terrible, I will never shed my weight" "I am so hopeless." Clara is already in a bad mood and devours a whole lot of donuts during the staff meeting. Sometimes your emotional eating and mood are directly related to your thoughts. The moment you realize that even though you have no control over a stressful situation, you can control the flood of negative and self-defeating thoughts, there is a higher chance of overcoming your emotional eating. Like I discussed earlier, in other to overcome this is to become aware of what you are thinking and the way you are feeling. Whenever you feel the urge to turn to food for comfort, you can whip out your journals and write down your thoughts. You will be amazed at how critical, harsh, and judgmental your thoughts are.

Replacing self-defeating thoughts

Self-defeating thoughts are usually triggered by situations that cause shame, anger, hurt, fear, and disappointment. There are ways to catch self-defeating thoughts and replacing them with non-judgmental and objective ones.

Step 1: Catch

Write down what you are thinking and feeling about your situation in a journal. Pick out the most troubling you have and work on it.

Step 2: Replace

Replace this thought with a non-judgmental one that is equally true. It might be hard to change deep-seated beliefs that you have held for a lifetime. This will require a lot of attention and dedication. It takes a lot of energy to manage your emotions. When you are having unpleasant emotions before you turn to food for comfort, stop to examine your thought, and pick out the most troubling one, replace them with empowering new thoughts. Creating empowering thoughts is often challenging because sometimes they don't feel true right away, and they may not be comforting. Patience is the key to this process.

For example, Carrie just spent time with her neighbor, where she talked non-stop about how slim she was and how her workout session is helping her get back in shape after childbirth. Carrie thought to herself, "Why is it hard for me to shed my weight?" "I'm a big fat failure."

Carrie can replace her thoughts with this, "When I take baby steps and set realistic goals about the pace at which I shed my weight, I can accomplish them."

Ways of creating empowering thoughts

When creating empowering thoughts, keep them simple, short, and in the present tense. Avoid using statements like "I will do……, sometimes in future".

Make these thoughts unconditional. Use a statement like "I can…."

Phrase these thoughts in a way that implies you are doing it rather than what you are not doing; for example, you say, "I will say loving things about myself" instead of "I will not say negative things to myself anymore.

Try thinking of neutral, non-judgmental thoughts, if you can't think of energizing ones. For example, "my stomach is big and unattractive" can be replaced with "my stomach is in the right proportion to my body."

Have gratitude thoughts that make you value what you have. Example "my arm is too fat," you can have. "I'm grateful for having strong arms that serve me well."

Think of comfort words you will say to a loved one that will help see a situation in a new way.

When you don't have enough time to think-up empowering words, go with neutral thoughts. Empowering thoughts restore optimism and believe in one's self and urges you to take action.

Recognizing your Hunger and fullness signal

The amount of energy required for metabolism by your body is regulated by appetite, and it varies from person to person. Chronic dieting has taught many overeaters over the years to be afraid of their hunger. Skipping or trying to control your meal or the amount of food you take disconnects you from your body. Many chronic dieters develop creative ways to ignore their hunger. They don't even know what it feels like to be hungry. This creates a disconnection with their bodies. Hunger can be felt through physical symptoms such as a decrease in energy level, decrease in the ability to concentrate, faintness, irritability, and headache. It can be a rumbling of your stomach. These signals tell us that it is time to provide your body with food. Hunger is a wonderful sign that our body is functioning properly; it is nature's way of ensuring our survival. Once we begin to eat, the hunger sensation begins to fade, and we near satiation, we quickly lose interest in the food, and the satisfaction derived from the taste, aroma, and flavor becomes reduced. But sometimes we experience false hunger which can be caused by the sight of food or its aroma. For example, I'm bored, am going to eat to keep myself busy. Also eat when running or in front of the T.V, compromise our ability to pick up our fullness signals. Your body has a way of regulating your weight, although these vary from one person to another. You will notice that you feel hungrier sometimes like when you exercise, a few days to your period. Your hunger should be dealt with according to the signal your body gives you. If you are the type that doesn't get hungry till late morning, wait till then before taking your meal, even though you have been taught to eat early breakfast. When you are experiencing true hunger, pick whatever food that looks good to you. Giving yourself a free choice of what to eat will reduce any sense of restriction and deprivation. When you are restricting yourself to the type of food to eat, there is a high chance you might overeat the food you wanted. Having cravings is normal as long as it disappeared after you have eaten, persistent craving might be an indication of emotional appetite. By now, we all know that emotional hunger feels like physical hunger. If you are not sure whether what you are feeling is true physical hunger, you can ask yourself whether you ate enough throughout yesterday, and today, if the answer is no, then what you are feeling is physical hunger even if you just ate a big meal. Your body might be telling you that you did not get enough calories and nutrients for it to function. You can have a light snack or fruit if it is late in the night. Then eat a good breakfast the next morning. If you did eat enough yesterday and today, but you are still hungry, try a light snack, but if the hunger persists, it might be an emotional one. Set limits for yourself by consciously allowing yourself a few bites of your forbidden food.

I will be answering some question that might come to your mind when listening to your hunger

What if there is no food around and I'm hungry: when you pay attention to hunger cues, you can anticipate your hunger. If this happens to you, you can cultivate the habit of carrying light snacks with you.

What if I have a lunch engagement or get together and am not hungry: this may be because you choose to eat before your hunger signal, or it is not yet time for your body to feel physical hunger. You can decide to eat a small amount of food or just munch on a light snack.

I am eating all the time: eating mini-meal many times per day helps you maintain your satisfaction and energy level. Many overeaters often eat large and fattier meals to carry them throughout the day, especially those with a fast metabolism; they find it stressful to keep eating mini food all the time. Your body takes this as a signal to store for the less raining days. It will rapidly store these calories in the form of fat. For those with slow body metabolism with milder hunger signals, they go without eating throughout the day and then overeat during the night. Often, when they start eating, they find it difficult to stop; this can be an indication that there is an imbalance with their appetite-stimulating and suppressing hormone as a result of irregularities in the way they eat, causing them to overeat.

What if I feel like eating even when I am not hungry: you eat for multiple reasons, and it has been established that not all hunger is truly physical. At times, the hunger you are experiencing is as a result of you wanting to distract yourself from a particular unpleasant emotion. You might find it unpleasant when you no longer make food a source of comfort and pleasure. Perhaps you have a negative emotion surfacing; you don't know how to deal with these emotions, try practicing inner conversation, or employ some of the emotional distress tools.

Recognizing your fullness signal

Fullness is an important signal developed to prevent us from overeating, becoming fat and sluggish. Generally, after about 15-20 min after we have begun eating, our stretch receptors will send a subtle signal that we have had enough. Stretch receptors are embedded in the stomach. They are designed to send us a signal telling us when we are full. If we ignore the signal being sent by the stretch receptors, it will send a louder signal. To stop eating when we feel this signal or immediately after the signal, we need to practice intuitive eating i.e., being mindful of this signal

How to carry out mindful eating

Intuitive eating is based on mindfulness meditation. It involves carefully noticing all the sensations you feel when you eat. The steps below will help you understand intuitive eating.

- Settle in a quiet and comfortable place
- Serve yourself a normal amount of your pleasure food
- Take time to admire and appreciate its visual appearance

Put it into your mouth and take time to describe the texture and appearance

What flavor can you detect?

Tasting food this way involves using all your senses, and it also gives pleasure

Tips for applying mindful eating

Eat only when you are hungry: mindful eating gives room for eating anything, you must feel real physical hunger before you eat

Take pleasure in your food: eating is one of the pleasures of life, take time to appreciate what you are eating.

Eat to satisfy true physical hunger and nothing more: do not rush your food, savor your food, this way you can easily recognize when you are full.

Zero guilt: mindful eating does not ban food; you can treat yourself to helpful pastries and not feel guilty about it. Guilt lowers your self-esteem and can result in food cravings.

Don't delay your meal until you are too hungry: this makes you lose control and overeat

Learn to trust yourself: if you cultivate self-trust, your hunger and fullness signal becomes more and more obvious to you.

Always stay hydrated: Thirst is a powerful biological signal, drinking an adequate amount of water keeps us hydrated and helps our signal to function properly.

Social gatherings and functions can create an avenue for overeating because of the abundance of food available. You can tune in on the signal your body is sending you and deciding when to stop. Treat yourself like a parent watching over a child at a party. The parent pays attention to what the child is eating. You can also apply this to yourself.

Also, you can try practicing the following social rules:

Be conscious and mindful of what you are eating: avoid unconsciously grabbing food and snacks by noticing and carefully selecting what you would like to eat

Stick to only one helping or plate: after you have eaten a plateful, do not go back for a second serving unless you are truly and physically hungry. Pay attention to your fullness level, once your body has given it fullness signal, move away from the food area.

Stop after three bites of dessert: Do not take more than three helpings of a desert in a function. When you are tempted to take more, leave the area or pass the desert to someone else. Remind yourself that it is easy to overeat and be tempted. And even if you do overeat, that does not mean it has ruined all your progress as long as you don't do these always, you are good to go.

Embracing your body wisdom

Sometimes, we view our body as our enemies, especially if you have been struggling with your weight for most of your life, whereas our body is our first warning system, especially when we are dealing with emotions that are serving as a trigger for our emotional eating. When you experience negative emotions about your body can result in a disconnection between you and your body. Some of this might be a result of the accumulation of past hurtful experiences often from our childhood. By connecting with your body, you can tap into its ability to heal itself.

Learn how to love your body image

Body image is the way you picture your body in your mind. When you don't have a positive image of your body in your mind, it indicates that emotional distress or depression. And this plays a major role in maintaining your emotional eating. Having a poor body image leads to you judging yourself based only on your looks. The society is not making it easy for people in bigger bodies as they view having a slim body as the criteria for beauty. We let society get to us about our body image. They generally criticize people that are not corresponding with the cultural standard of thinness. The next time you want to compare or judge your body, why not choose someone with a less conventional body type living healthily or better place more priority on your body function which is often forgotten in a bid to compare our body with the more conventional types. Even though the media and the western world project, the image of an ideal body type, some experience in our childhood can also be the cause of this problem. Your parent relationship with you as a child has a direct impact on your social development, emotions, thoughts, and expectations in the future. Have you ever wondered why this media projection affects you deeply? This is because you might have suffered rejection as a child, especially from your parents. When you are focusing on a lot of hurt feelings and emotions from the past, it will be difficult to connect with your body.

Body disconnection

When you are not satisfied with your body, it can cause you to disconnect from it, such that when you look into the mirror, you tend to see only your face and ignore your whole body, or you avoid taking a look at the mirror altogether. You where loose cloth to avoid dealing with your discomfort and dissatisfaction with your body size or shape. This makes you lose touch with the sensation and signal given by your body. If you examine it, body disconnection is probably the reason why you want to rigidly control your body shape and size with extreme dieting and excessive exercise. When you are constantly checking for fats in your body, pinching yourself for fatness or constantly weighing your body to check your weight is a sign that you are disconnected from your body.

Practice mindfulness. Address the negative thought you have about your body, and finally, learn to trust yourself and your body wisdom.

Learn how to respect your body

Accept your body the way it is; this has been discussed earlier in this chapter. Respect your body so you can feel better about yourself, practice self-compassion in a way that shows you respect your body and cares for it. Being too vigilant over your body leads to you worrying about your body. This, in turn, create emotions that trigger eating. Have you ever thought about the fact that dwelling on your imperfect body image did not help you get leaner? Respecting your body means catering for its daily needs and treating it with care and dignity. If you are a person that has been using food to deal with emotions over time, your present body image might be the result of the way you cared for your body. Respecting your body is an important factor in becoming a mindful eater.

How to respect your body

Your body has some basic needs that must be met, such as feeding, bathing, and comfortably dressing your body. Respecting your body is an easy concept to understand, but it can be very difficult to practice. The following tools will help you establish a new relationship with your body.

Get comfortable with your body

Do not wear clothes that serve as a constant reminder of the way your body looks. Yes, it will be difficult to show respect to your body, but you will overcome it with time. These clothes serve as a reminder of what you want to be. Simply changing your underwear to the more comfortable one goes a long way to make you feel good about yourself.

Change the way you assess your body

It has been discovered that repeatedly weighing yourself to check your body weight leads to constantly worrying about your body weight. This makes it difficult to accept your present body. My solution to this is to stop weighing yourself. Using a piece of cloth smaller than your size and trying it on daily can make you feel bad about your body. Get rid of it and start practicing mindful eating, accepting your hunger, self –compassion and reframing your thoughts

Stop comparing your body to others

People, upon entering a room, start comparing their bodies with the rest of the crowd. They begin a game of "who has the biggest body in the room." They envy other people's shapes, "she must work-out a lot if only I have her shape." You can't judge other people by their shape and assumed they earned it; you must know we are all different from one another, and the way we respond to situations and emotions are different. Playing the body-check game results in more dissatisfaction with your body.

Stop body criticism

Stop focusing on your imperfect body; every time you do this, you become self-conscious and start worrying about your body.

Get adequate sleep

Lack of adequate sleep usually leads to irritation and crankiness, with overeating and weight gain as a common side effect. Have you noticed that you are always hungry once you don't get enough sleep? Adequate sleep is one of the important ways of regulating body weight and health. Many people who are sleep deprived often turn to food to fill up their depleted energy reserve. Increasing evidence has suggested that a lack of sleep has multiple effects on the body, especially on body weight. Sleep is an important biological active time where a lot of activities such as maintenance, repair, and detoxification occurs. Disruption of this active time as an effect on a lot of bodily functions such as cognitive function, hormonal balance, and immunity. Chronic sleep deprivation results in anxiety, irritation, and depression. All these are a contributor to emotional eating. The research conducted by scientists has shown that when you get adequate sleep, you give your body a better chance of regulating your body chemicals. In other words, the more the adequate sleep you get, the better your body is at regulating the chemicals controlling your fullness and hunger. Also, long-term sleep deprivation interferes with the endocrine system of the body leading to increased insulin resistance. This disrupts the hormones that regulate your appetite. When you are sleep deprived, there is an increase in ghrelin, the hormone that makes you feel hungry, and a reduction in leptin the hormone that makes you feel full. Substances like caffeine and other nicotine can interfere with the production of the sleep-inducing hormone. Some certain foods can also interfere with your ability to get a night of restful sleep, for example, having a light carbohydrate snack can induce sleep because of the effect they have on the serotonin level why it is best to avoid heavy food before bedtime as this can lead to digestive disturbance. In addition to a heavy meal, low-level anxiety and stress can rob us of our sleep. When you Sometimes, we experience sleepless nights, it is normal, but when it becomes a regular experience, it is known as chronic insomnia. This can be caused by a physiological condition or just poor sleeping habits.

Adjust your sleeping habits if you find it difficult to get a restful sleep. For instance, you can try dimming the light in your room 1-2hours before bed; exposure to light, whether artificial or natural, stimulates the release of excitatory hormones, making it difficult for our body to unwind and fall asleep. Just as the body as a way of telling us when we are hungry and full, it also has a way of signaling us when it is time to rest and sleep. Long term and short term accumulation of sleeplessness may have a serious health implication.

Develop New Core Beliefs

Core beliefs are formed when we are young, while we were experiencing intense emotional upheaval and during the transition. It is defined as the basic belief we have about ourselves and others. In other words, it is the way you view yourself, other people, and the world in general. Core beliefs are things you accept as true without any question, and they determine the degree to which you view yourself as worthy, loved, and competent. It is connected to our primary needs, such as the need for love, safety, and trust. It is triggered when we are in a situation that is threatening to those primary needs or when we are coping with a situation that we are too inexperienced to handle.

A negative core belief is usually seen among individuals with an emotional eating disorder than people with no eating disorder. It is dangerous to your self-acceptance and self-esteem. Addressing a negative core belief is important because if left unchecked might make it difficult for you to stop unhealthy behaviors. A negative core belief is an important factor in the cause and maintenance of emotional eating. Negative core beliefs can lead to compulsive behaviors such as overeating and bingeing.

Core beliefs can also be formed if you are neglected during your childhood, especially children who grow up in a home where there a lot of rules devised to suppress, ignore, and control their feelings. You know when you are in your core belief when you are experiencing the same body sensation, thought, and emotions anytime you are behaving from one of your primary core belief. For example, a person who fears failure can work about ninety hours per week in an attempt to avoid failure. Most times, overworking backfires because they don't often neglect their body signal for rest and when the body shuts down and they are unable to work, their sense of failure is increased. This core belief can also be an indication of a persisting problem in your life, like reoccurring emotional eating and the inability to maintain a healthy weight. If your core belief is opposing your current goals and desire, it will be of great benefit to you if you can identify and change these core beliefs. Core beliefs not only affect your relationship with food, but it also affects the way you handle stress, your relationship with your body, and your relationship with others. Core belief impacts the way we perceive and interprets a situation; they affect the way we judge others and ourselves.

How to identify core beliefs

Identifying your core beliefs is the first step in changing them. The first step in identifying your core belief is developing an awareness of your thought. How to become aware of your thought has been discussed in the earlier part of this chapter. Core belief can be identified by using the downward arrow technique, which is following the pattern of your thought down to fundamental belief it came from. To start, bring to your mind a thought you have always had about yourself regularly like "I don't always get it right." Ask yourself, "What does it indicate about me."

Your answer should indicate something about you as a person like, "I'm scared of being a failure."

Then ask yourself again what it means about "what does this mean about me."

The answer can be "I lack motivation" or "I'm a failure."

Once your core issue has been identified, you can now start a self-conversion on how to deal with those beliefs.

How to change your core belief

Changing core beliefs is not an easy task. Core beliefs are some fundamental things we believe about ourselves. The first thing you need to do is change the perspective about things. Core beliefs are like dreams; when you are dreaming, they look real to you. This is the same for core belief. Changing your perspective is like waking up from a dream and facing the real reality.

You can practice letting go by following the steps below

Identifying your core beliefs and how it had served you when it first developed

Develop a new guiding principle

Pick an object that will be a symbol of your new guiding principle. The object could be a plant or a picture

Develop a skill to deal with your emotions.

Create a Support System

Having a support system is very important when it comes to emotional eating and weight management i.e., people who will love and encourage you. A support system serves as a source of positive encouragement and keeps you accountable. This is how a support group works, people in your support group don't scold you when you fail to meet your set of goals. Instead, they listen and make suggestions on how best they can support you in the future. Make sure to explain to them that you rely on them for support, and if the need arises for them to be firm with you, they should not hold back, but at the same time, it should be done in a gentle and corrective manner.

A grave mistake that can be committed by you is trying to manipulate your support group, this can backfire and jeopardize all your plans, and you need to be as honest as possible with them. Take note of what works for you, so that you can choose the right people for your support group. Some people prefer motivational talk and constructive confrontation, while some appreciate a strict approach. You can pick the one you are comfortable with and also remember you have to be flexible because the need might arise for you to change the approach.

Creating a support system at home

Home support depends on people who we live with and the people around us. They are the most familiar with our needs and the challenges we are facing. If your support system are members of your family and they are not too desirable, you can have a conversation with them and let them know how important it is for you to have them supporting you. If some of them want to sabotage your success, it is important to reduce the amount of time you spend with such people.

Here are some suggestions on how a home support group can work effectively

When you are tempted with food that is your triggers, or you want to use food to deal with a particular emotion, your support person can help devise a means to deal with such situations; they can say or do anything that will help you get past such episodes. They can create a distraction technique that will help you forget about food

When you are tempted to turn to food, talk to your support person, you can also ask your support person to move your trigger food to a place you are not aware of to keep you from being tempted by them.

Encourage your support group to ask when you need motivation, encouragement, or when you need reminders about your goals to eat healthily.

Here are a few questions that will help you communicate better with your support group

    How is my support system at home?

    What negative criticism am I telling myself?

    Why do I have this feeling?

    What works for your home support system when you are really in need of help?

How would I want my home support to work?

What amendment do I need to make as my needs change?

Creating a support system at work

If you are the type that spends a lot of time at your place of work, you might require their support just like it is at home, but in this case, only if you are comfortable with doing so. You can ask your co-workers for support, but this can be disastrous if you and your co-workers are not on the same wavelength. If this is happening, choose co-workers that will be on your side. Creating a work support system could be a huge success with strategies, awareness, and willingness. Develop questions that will help you communicate better with your support system at work. You can use the same approach for the home support group. Don't just assume that it is their responsibility to know what you are thinking. Have a good interaction with your support people; they can help you avoid situations whereby you are tempted to eat something unhealthy. They can also help with distraction strategies that will take your mind away from food. They can help remove high-risk food around you, motivate, encourage, and help you realize your goals. Like I discussed earlier, communicate your need to your support person or team. Let them know when to be firm with you or when to motivate you.

Here are a few strategies that can be used by you and your work support group.

Focus on your work. This is important because it keeps your mind from thinking about food

Prepare healthy food for lunch

Take lunch during your break

Always keep yourself hydrated with water

Do not keep sweets and snacks on your desk as this can be a source of temptation

If there are a birthday or retirement celebrations, go for the healthy options

Develop strategies to cope with overeating outside your home

Social Outings

Going to a restaurant, fast food, and other social events can pose a challenge to our goals. When we eat out, we presume we have no control over the preparation and the ingredients used in the preparation of the meal. For some people, eating out implies that they can abandon their food plan during this time. This can lead to self-defeating thoughts when we make a decision that is against our food plan. We make assumptions about how to behave and what to do when we are dining out, some even permit themselves to overeat. When in their homes, they follow their set of goals and rules, but a dinner or a party can be disastrous to them because they don't know how to control themselves beyond their homes. It is important to keep a journal because, most of the time, we don't remember what works for us when we are experiencing intense emotions; in other words, we don't remember the way we deal with these emotions. Always remember to write what works for you in your journal

Restaurants

In North America, value is placed not on quality alone but also on quantity; you need to make plans ahead of going to a restaurant to eat. When you are ordering in a restaurant, order for the smaller portion or half portion. If the restaurant does not agree with this, ask for a take-out container to come with your meal, this helps you to judge the amount of food you can eat before the body signals that you are full and also whatever you are not eating can be set aside in the container. When you do this, you will discover that you are not tempted to overeat. Some restaurants will tell you they don't have a smaller option, but you can just talk to a waitress to reduce the amount of food that will be served to you at the full price. This is a better and realistic option because eating a larger meal can trigger emotions like guilt and shame and a risk to your food plan.

Here are a few strategies to employ when dining in a restaurant

Make sure to call the restaurant the restaurant ahead of time for the menu so that you can decide on what to order ahead of time

If you are not sure about your ability to order food in front of other people, it is always wise to pre-order your food

If you are always tempted by what other people are ordering, you can always ask your companions or friend if you could place your order. This will prevent you from being by what others are eating.

When it comes to ordering of gravies and sauce in general, order them separately on the side so that you can control the number of gravies and sauce you take.

If the size of the meal is larger than what you needed, you can ask for another plate and divide the meal into two portions.

Fast food

In general, fast food restaurant serves food that is rich in sugar, fats, and carbohydrate. In fast-food restaurants, values are placed on quantity. When picking a fast food restaurant to dine out, pick the one that has safe and healthy options on their menu. One good trick to use in a fast food restaurant is to order a kid-size meal to give the advantage of small size; you can also go online to check the percentage and nutritional values of their menu ahead of time. Decide what will work for you before going to the fast-food restaurant. This saves your time and energy and prevents you from making bad decisions that will lead to guilt, shame, and feeling out of control. These feelings upset your planned goals and have a negative impact on your resolve of eating healthily.

Do not restrict yourself about going to a fast-food restaurant, rather make a smart decision that will make this enjoyable and pleasurable for you. Going to a fast food restaurant is inevitable, but you can choose food that is in order with your daily eating plan. Remember to practice mindful eating (describe earlier this chapter). Choosing the menu and following through with what you have on your eating plans motivates and encourages you to practice healthier eating.

Buffets

Buffets are often billed as "All you can eat!" The buffet table can sometimes be overwhelming. Most of the time, what comes to mind during a buffet is what best choice can be made, how do you get your money worth. The last choice is how the content of the buffet table fits into your daily eating plan. In a buffet, there are so many options and tempting dishes. This can create a headache when we want to make a decision on what to eat. If you are scared of buffets. Don't go to one until you are comfortable with choosing the food that fits into your eating plan. Don't be too hung up on the cost; believe you are paying for the experience. When taking part in a buffet, survey the spread for choices that will fit accordingly to your plan. If the buffet is in a friend's home, ask to be seated far away from the buffet table. Select a smaller plate if that is available, and if not, make sure your food is within the inner circle of a dinner plate.

An important thing to note: resist the temptation to go back for a second serving, take your time to eat, and savor your food. Select fruit for dessert instead of pastries.

Vacation

Vacation is like an avenue for dinning three times a day. Eating during vacation is not a big deal as long as you have a plan.

What to do when you are on vacation

Find out about the food available in your vacation spot, their health implications, if they fit into your eating plan.

Fill a cooler with healthy snacks, vegetables, and fruits.

Make finding of the food offered by your motel or hotel. Ask if they have healthy menu alternatives.

Always practice mindful eating and remember to eat in moderation.

Conclusion

The journey was long, but you have finally reached the end. Hopefully, your emotional eating/ food addiction problem has also met its end. Each chapter in the book had a purpose in the journey and touched the aspects necessary for the redefinition of your relationship with food.

Chapter one defined the problem (emotional eating and food addiction) and went on to help you understand that some of those random eating and rewarding habits were dangerous. It also differentiated emotional eating from food addiction. It's a popular misconception that both habits are one and the same, but the differences between both were fully explained in the chapter.

After diagnosing the problem in the first chapter, the second chapter defined what the normal relationship between man and food should be. It talked about the reasons why men should eat, the differences between physical hunger and emotional hunger, the emotional eating triggers, and

Chapter three dived into the impacts of emotional eating on health. It listed and explained the different disorders associated with food. It discussed the side effects of the overeating caused by emotional eating and food addiction, the type of people plagued by emotional eating and food addiction, and the manner in which the habit is showcased in adults and children.

Chapter four, when to the root of the problem by defining emotions and explaining the chemical processes involved in the creation of emotions. It explained how the emotions we feel are related to food, the roles emotions have to play in our daily activities, the types of emotions we feel, and the mechanics of how the brain makes us feel them. The logic behind explaining the creation of emotions in the chapter is that the more you understand how your emotions are created, the more you have power over them.

The power-packed fifth chapter of this book was about helping you create the right mindset to overcome your problem. Being the longest and most important chapter of the book, it challenged the readers to change their food habits by participating in activities that are healthy and calming to the soul. It covered everything that had to do with mental control over emotions and also taught the reader how to respect their bodies.

You're finally done with the book and must have learned multiple strategies to help you cope and manage your food addiction and emotional eating. Just as the title of the book says, this is the end to your "Lifelong addiction." However, reading this book is not the end. You have to follow it up with strict discipline over your eating habits. Without discipline, you may find yourself back to square one, rereading the book or other materials to end your addiction.

Resources

www.positivepsychology.com

www.verywellmind.com

www.psychalive.org

American Psychiatric Association

www.Reddeltaproject.com

www.Mayoclinic.org

www.bulimia.com

www.medicinenet.com

www.britannica.com

www.imotions.com

www.psychologydiscussion.net

www.verywell.com

www.parentingforbrain.com

www.apibhs.com

www.researchgate.net

www.explorable.com

https://www.disabled-world.com/fitness/nutrition/

https://www.healthline.com/nutrition/10-super-healthy-high-fat-foods#section10

https://www.helpguide.org/harvard/vitamins-and-minerals.htm

https://www.precisionnutrition.com/all-about-vitamins-minerals

https://medium.com/macrokitchen/the-top-5-functions-of-fat-in-your-diet-3530585271a8

https://www.healthline.com/health/food-nutrition/six-essential-nutrients#protein

https://www.scientificamerican.com/article/why-does-your-stomach-gro/ Emotional Intelligence 2.0 by Jean Greaves Travis Bradberry

The emotional brain by Joseph Ledoux

Emotional Freedom by Judith Orloff, M.D

www.ingramcontent.com/pod-product-compliance
Lightning Source LLC
Chambersburg PA
CBHW070053120526
44588CB00033B/1423